FIC Robinson
Robinson, Kathleen.
    Heaven's only daughter.

Heaven's Only Daughter

ALSO BY KATHLEEN ROBINSON

DOMINIC

HEAVEN'S ONLY DAUGHTER

KATHLEEN ROBINSON

St. Martin's Press New York

This novel is a work of fiction. All of the events, characters, names and places depicted in this novel are entirely fictitious or are used fictitiously. No representation that any statement made in this novel is true or that any incident depicted in this novel actually occurred is intended or should be inferred by the reader.

HEAVEN'S ONLY DAUGHTER. Copyright © 1993 by Kathleen Robinson. All rights reserved. Printed in the United States of America. No part of this book may be used or reproduced in any manner whatsoever without written permission except in the case of brief quotations embodied in critical articles or reviews. For information, address St. Martin's Press, 175 Fifth Avenue, New York, N.Y. 10010.

Editor: Sandra D. McCormack
Production Editor: David Stanford Burr
Design: Judith A. Stagnitto

Library of Congress Cataloging-in-Publication Data
Robinson, Kathleen.
    Heaven's only daughter / Kathleen Robinson.
       p. cm.
    ISBN 0-312-09304-7
    1. Rome—History—Honorius, 395–423—Fiction. I. Title.
PS3568.O28919H4   1993
813'.54—dc20   93-15063
                                        CIP

First Edition: August 1993

10 9 8 7 6 5 4 3 2 1

For my lovely niece,
Karla Michelle

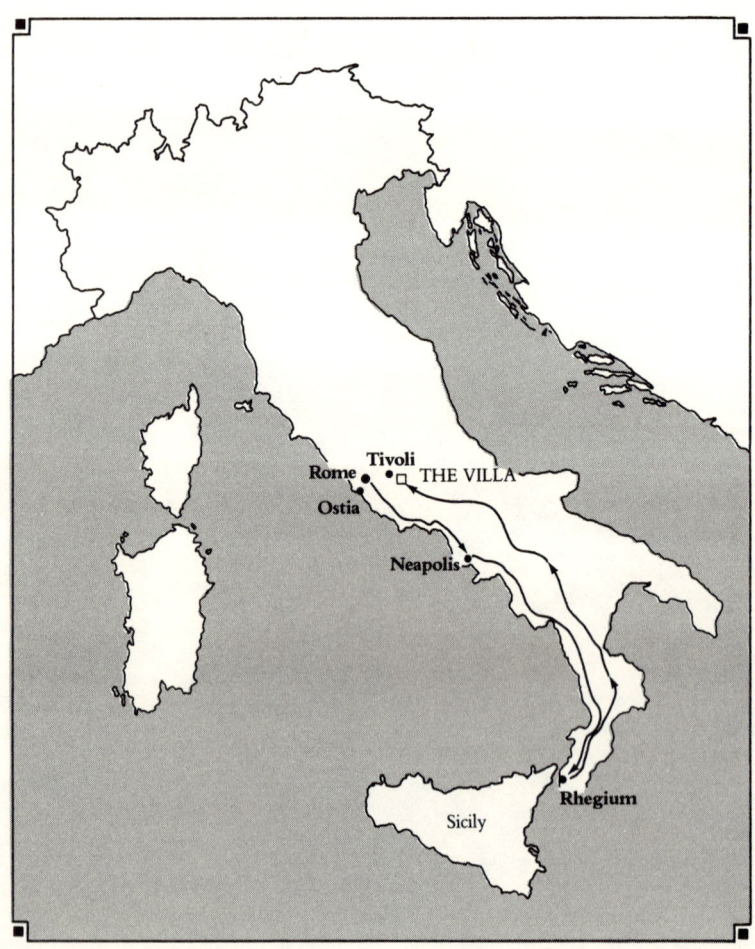

Heaven's Only Daughter

In the summer of 410 A.D., barbarian Goths
overran the City of Rome. When they departed,
they took as hostage the Emperor's half-sister,
Imperial Princess Galla Placidia.
Naturally, the lady objected . . .

1

IMPERIAL PRINCESS Galla Placidia was glad she did not believe in omens. Her first official act had been to sign her cousin's death warrant. Now her first official appearance was her cousin's execution here on the terrace before the Great Palace.

Beneath the terrace the Circus Maximus was a sea of colorful cloaks, tunics, and scarves, but to the Imperial Princess—Dia to everyone who knew her—they were but a blur of chattering motion.

She was gathering her courage to face the consequences of those few seconds in which she had scratched her signature on a piece of new parchment.

She had not wanted to be here, but they convinced her it was necessary—the Princeps and the Prefect—to show that one of the Imperial family listened to the citizens of Rome, that the Senate and the Imperials stood together on this decision.

Her nurse Elpidia put it even more bluntly. "You signed your name to that paper, lovey. Easy enough to sign your name and forget it, but her ladyship's life was on that paper—though I don't doubt she earned her just deserts honestly, mind you—but if you claim the authority to end a life, then you ought to be able to face it straight on. Show them what you're made of, Mistress Imperial Princess; show them the daughter of Emperor Theodosius and Empress Galla is no coward. Give 'em pause to know Galla Placidia is to be reckoned with, or they'll never take you seriously."

Pidi was right, she knew. They would never take her seriously if she hid behind her palace walls. They would think she was a coward—she *would* be a coward—and for the daughter and granddaughter of emperors that was intolerable.

This still autumn morning Dia wore an ostentatious gown with purple and gold embroidery and her heavy mantle, its borders encrusted with pearls, amethysts, and emeralds in a floral design.

She was hot and uncomfortable, but held her head high, and somewhat stiffly, to keep her jeweled coiffure in place.

Dia had prayed half the night. She prayed not for guidance; the decision was made, the act done. The laws of the Empire must be upheld; treason was punishable by death; the throne must maintain authority. She prayed for forgiveness, for understanding, for peace of mind, for courage to face this day.

Still, Placidia was unprepared for the sight of her cousin Serena slowly, carefully, descending the palace steps, wearing a mourning dress of shining white, leaning on Cassandra, her physician. Serena walked unsteadily toward the center of the terrace but drew back when the scream of the crowd in the Circus cheered her appearance. For a better view, spectators in the tiers directly below the terrace ran out onto the dirt track, craning their necks and jeering at the woman in white.

Serena looked terrified, Dia thought with a pang of guilt, and she wished for a moment that it was not too late to change her mind. But as Serena's gaze fell upon her, her cousin's expression became one of withering scorn. She stopped and faced her royal cousin, putting all the bitter hatred she felt in her icy grey eyes.

Dia forced herself to meet Serena's eyes.

I will survive this horrible spectacle. Serena will not.

Dia looked away first, unable to face down her cousin's accusing gaze. Serena gripped Cassandra's arm with renewed desperation.

With growing dread Dia watched Serena stagger toward the front of the terrace, where awaited the executioners. The crowd went wild with jubilation. When Bishop Innocent approached to bestow upon her a final benediction, Serena's hard grey eyes met him with a look of pure venom.

The resolution of the Senate was read aloud, with careful note made of Placidia's signature.

She would escape no responsibility for this day, nor did she wish to. Dia steeled her nerves with a lifetime of court training, setting her face stiffly into an expression of Imperial gravity.

The executioners bound Serena's hands behind her back. With bitter disdain, Serena stared straight ahead, above the heads in the highest tier in the Circus, across the City to the sea of grey clouds draining the blue from the sky.

The silken cord snaked around Serena's throat. Serena crumpled to her knees, fear draining all the strength from her.

Dia clenched her fists, trembling.

Behind the kneeling woman, the executioner twisted the cord, and as her breath was slowly cut off, a cry of rasping terror wrenched from Serena's open mouth, a sound soon lost in excited cheers from the stands.

Dia longed to cover her face but knew the daughter of Theodosius could allow herself no escape from the horrible scene.

Serena struggled wildly, trying to fling herself left and right; the relentlessly tightening cord kept her from falling. Her eyes bulged in terror; her face was ghastly.

Dia clenched her jaws, dug her fingernails into her palms. *Mother of God, let it be over quickly.*

Serena's blue face contorted into a hideous, soundless scream as she flopped like a rabbit caught in a noose.

Dia felt a sick horror rising in her throat. With all her will she forced her eyes to remain on Serena's dying struggles.

Finally, finally, Serena's legs stopped thrashing and she lay still, dangling from the silken cord, her blue-black face fallen to one side, her bulging eyes staring across the tiers of the Circus and its scarf-waving, cheering throng.

Placidia turned away, gulping in huge, gasping breaths, tears blinding her eyes, a silent scream of her own forcing its way up her throat. Hands pressed to her chest, to her heart, she fought the feeling that she would explode.

Slowly, with desperate dignity, she departed the terrace. She did not vomit; she did not scream; she did not cry. But in the hollow vestibule of the Great Palace she beat both fists against a frescoed wall until searing pain shot up through her arms to her shoulders—until Thalia and Dulcie pulled her back and held her trembling between them.

She could not shut out the vision of Serena's dying struggles, her distorted face, her dead eyes. Dia wondered if she would ever be able to see anything but the terrible sight of Serena's last gasps for breath.

The next morning, beneath the weak sunrise of a bleak and dreary dawn, a steady drizzle fell upon the armor, helmets, and spears of Alaric the Goth's barbarian army camped before every gate of the City.

2

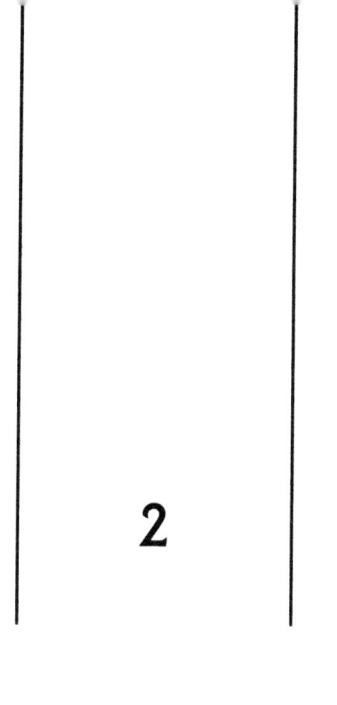

DIA FELT she would have lost her mind, if not her soul, in those horrible months following Serena's execution if it had not been for Elpidia. The sleepless nights, the dreams, sudden tears, her inability to eat, and long vigils kneeling before the gentle figure of Mary which occupied a niche in the atrium—all this was countered by Pidi's practical, worldly wisdom.

"Goes with the purple," Pidi would say, or, "Treason's got to be discouraged, or everyone would be at it." Sometimes in the night she held the restless, weeping princess in her arms and whispered, "You did the right thing, lovey, the *only* thing. I know it's hard, bless you, being the one, but I expect God chose you because you *do* have a heart; I expect he's teaching you wisdom and strength in his own way. Mark my words, Dia, the Lord's got his own plans for you."

The vision of Serena's death struggles did fade with time, until it seemed more like a vivid nightmare she had once upon a time. A year later it was as though Serena had never been. Dia was in charge of her own properties now, estates and investments scattered across the Empire, but little good they did her, trapped in Rome as she was. The roads were unsafe with the barbarians raiding about as they pleased, setting a bad example for peasants and slaves who saw the profit in banditry. Communication to anywhere outside the City was shaky at best, since only one in ten messengers ever made it past the Goths.

The hated Goths! Just one year after their first siege of Rome, they had blockaded the City again. Again the people were starving—scarcely a living animal, no stray cat or dog or goose, survived within the walls—even horses had not escaped the ravenous demands of the trapped populace. Dia hugged her beloved cat to her breast, feeling the deep purr of life contained in that warm little body.

"Treason!" Imperial Princess Galla Placidia spun to face the old statesman draped meticulously in the white, red-trimmed toga of a Senator, her eyes flashing like brittle blue-green topaz. "What you contemplate is no less than treason, Attalus. I suggest you reconsider."

"It is already accomplished, nobilissima," former First Senator Priscus Attalus told her mildly. "The Senate has voted."

"The Senate!" Placidia took an angry pace toward him, gold threadwork in her deep aquamarine gown glittering in the sullen light of the oil lamps. "The Senate," she told him imperiously, "does not *vote* on who shall be Emperor."

"Nevertheless, it has now."

"I cannot believe this. That you should allow the Senate to go so far astray as to commit high treason, and put *your* neck to the blade." Her eyes narrowed. "You, of all people, Attalus, know the punishment for such an act."

"I know," said Priscus Attalus, briefly bowing his head, his high forehead age-speckled. He had thought of this. Tomorrow he would be proclaimed Emperor—if the Senate's plan failed, his life would be forfeit, his head be flung from Tarpeian Rock.

"Then why? Why do you do it?"

"I do it for Rome, nobilissima. For Rome and for the Empire."

"You name yourself Emperor at the instigation of Alaric the Goth, the most deadly enemy Rome has ever known, and you have the gall to stand here and tell me it is for the good of the *Empire?*"

"I do *not* name myself Emperor." Priscus Attalus was becoming annoyed. "The *Senate* has chosen me by a nearly unanimous vote to don the purple—"

"Then the entire Senate is guilty of treason."

"—and set myself to the task of saving Rome from sure destruction—a task which the present Emperor neglects to our peril."

"Yet *you* would save it by collusion with our enemies—with that *savage* who calls himself a king!"

"That savage, nobilissima, has Rome in a stranglehold and is perfectly capable of choking the life out of this City."

"I suppose I am deposed also."

"You are still nobilissima," he said gently. "The Senate has no quarrel with you, only with your brother."

She looked up sharply. "And is that supposed to mollify me, Attalus, into condoning this travesty?"

Attalus sighed. "The Senate has acted, Princess; whether you condone the decision is immaterial."

Dia stared at him wonderingly. "Then why are you here, Attalus? Why do they send you to me?"

"No one sends me, nobilissima." Priscus Attalus spoke gently. "I thought you had a right to know, er"—the old statesman cleared his throat nervously—"how things stand." He was finding this difficult; against his better judgment he had allowed himself to become somewhat fond of the Imperial Princess. "There is more to it than—"

"More!" She was incredulous. "What more can there be?

You and the Senate have already committed the gravest treason. Honorius—*Emperor* Honorius—is the only lawful sovereign over the Western Empire, and no vote of the Senate can change that."

"Your brother," Attalus snapped in retort, "is no more competent to be Emperor than a cockerel!"

Dia gasped, her shapely lips rounded in open-mouthed astonishment.

"Do you know he is a matter of jest among the people, Princess? Even his own officers say that the only Roma which Honorius Augustus recognizes is his pet *chicken* by the same name!"

Dia was speechless. No, she had not known Honorius was the butt of such jests; such things were not spoken within her hearing. The worst of it was, she suspected the jest came uncomfortably close to the truth.

"Rome is in grave danger, nobilissima. *You* are in grave danger, and where is the Emperor? Where are the legions? We have been abandoned to our fate, and you, his own sister, he has abandoned with us. I propose to take up the purple and the diadem and do everything within my power to save the people of Rome from slow starvation by a barbaric king and an incompetent Emperor!"

This aged usurper to her brother's throne stood before her fired with courage and conviction. How could this be happening, she wondered, that from the most noble of motives—if he spoke the truth—he could contemplate the most treasonous of actions? She must persuade him to give up this fool's errand.

"Honorius will have your head for this," Dia told him levelly.

"Very well," Attalus answered just as levelly, "he is welcome to this old head. I look forward to it, since he will find it necessary to free the City to remove this head."

They glared at each other, the flushed young Imperial Princess and the iron-eyed former First Senator, former Prefect of Rome, now usurper Emperor.

Dia finally spoke. "I shall go to Ravenna and speak to

Honorius myself. He will listen to me if I explain the situation. I can persuade him to do something."

Attalus was shaking his head.

"Oh, I promise *I* shall return, Attalus, but with the Roman Legions at my back."

"You cannot go, nobilissima."

"Why not? You can arrange safe passage with your friend Alaric, can you not? You can make him see the advantage of it."

"It is one of Alaric's express demands that you remain within the City."

"What? His demand?" She was on her feet now, staring at him in horror. "Am I a hostage, then?"

The old Senator cleared his throat.

"Am I his hostage?"

"Not precisely."

Dia felt for her chair and sank down in a daze. Her voice sounded far away and very faint even to herself.

"What, precisely, do you mean?"

"Alaric feels that if you remain in the City he has more leverage with the Emperor."

For the first time real fear touched her. "How very strange of him, Attalus, since you claim that *you* are Emperor just now."

"He doesn't want an army marching out of Ravenna to dispute my claim."

"How very thoughtful of Alaric. You have a treaty with him, then?"

"Yes. It goes into effect when I am invested—tomorrow."

Dia's voice shook a little. "And I am to be a prisoner in the City?"

"Yes." Why did he find it so hard to say this to her? "The Prefect guard is even now replacing your own Protectors and Scholarians. I am sorry, nobilissima."

For a long moment Dia could not speak. She felt as if a

tremendous weight pressed down upon her chest, making each breath come hard and painful. At last her eyes focused on Attalus. Her lower lip trembled when she spoke.

"I suppose I should be grateful you didn't agree to hand me over to him outright."

The grey head nodded briefly. "I refused him that, Princess."

Dia twisted her hands together. So the barbarian had demanded her as a hostage after all. And Priscus Attalus had refused.

"But I am under guard in my palace?"

"In my custody. But I assure you—"

"For how long, Attalus?"

He hesitated again. "I wish I could say, nobilissima. The course of events is . . . uncertain. Perhaps it depends on whether Alaric gets what he wants for his people."

"I see," Dia said faintly, but even now she touched upon a note of irony in her next question. "May I ask, if it's any of my business, being merely the hostage in this case, just what you have promised Alaric when you are Emperor?"

Attalus hesitated a long moment, facing those sea-green eyes in the youthful face pale with strain. "I will appoint him Master of Both Armies."

"My God! Are you insane?"

"It was part of his demand." Attalus hesitated again, sighed, and went on. "His brother will be Count of the Domestic Horse."

"Holy Mother of God." She clenched her fingers tightly in her lap and stared at him. "What have you done to us, Attalus?"

"What your brother should have done. I will draw up a treaty granting land to the Goths as loyal federates of the Empire."

"You cannot do that without support from the legions—you have no army—"

"The Goths are my army; Alaric is my Master General."

"Our enemy!"

"He says he wants only peace."

"And you believe him?" Dia was incredulous.

"I have to believe him. Peace with Alaric is our only hope."

Sadly she shook her head. "I fear you have made a terrible mistake, Attalus. From the Goths you can expect only treachery."

3

ATAWULF, THE Bold Wolf, watched the sky. A glimmer of stars broke through the black vault overhead, over the City, but the flash and play of lightning illuminated the huge clouds rumbling and roiling toward the walls. Thunder, like the growling of wolves deep in their throats, accompanied the racing fields of light, as though the black clouds roared at each other in gigantic bad temper, as though Titans tossed bright fire back and forth, as though the old god Thunar rumbled across the sky in his chariot, the great wheels showering the heavens with white-hot flames.

Bold Wolf wondered if he believed in omens.

He looked to Alaric, and in the eerie play of ghostly light across his foster brother's face Atawulf saw the lips drawn back in that familiar grin, the glittering blue eyes fixed on the gate.

Alaric clearly did not believe in omens. Or, if he did, he took this storm as an omen for Rome: *Beware, the Goths are upon you!*

A closer, brighter flash of lightning in the sky, followed by a louder clash of thunder, caused Atawulf's restless mount to stamp and lay back his ears, roll back his eyes. Perhaps the Red Demon, in all this readiness for war, mistook the storm for the sounds of battle; or perhaps the thunder and lightning spooked him, though the Goths' animals had been through all manner of storms, usually unsheltered. Atawulf held him in check and smoothed the muscled neck; the stamping quieted, though it had gone unheard, the steed's hooves being muffled with leather socks—as were all the horses' hooves.

He could scarcely believe he would soon be riding into Rome. Could it be a trap? He shrugged the notion away. Under cover of this black night, ten thousand Gothic cavalry gathered in long formation behind him, like a creaking leather-and-iron centipede on hooves.

If that gate opened, Atawulf knew, no force on Earth could halt them.

Suddenly, metal shrieked on metal, and the shadowed gate swung outward, slowly. He briefly glimpsed the form of a woman in the narrow opening, but she disappeared at once. Now men appeared from within, pushing the gate open speedily, until a gaping hole lay wide open in the wall of Rome.

The Gothic cavalry did not charge into the dark womb of Rome at a gallop. Alaric spoke briefly to a captain at the gates; then, at a walk, the war-horses of the Goths stepped four abreast through the Salarian Gate.

Not until a goodly number of his cavalry had entered the dark and deserted street, the sounds of their passage obscured in the growing bellow and rage of thunder, did Alaric signal to light their torches from those in the gatehouse.

When the soldiers from the gate were mounted to guide them into the heart of the City, Alaric raised his torch aloft, yellow-orange flame dancing off his helm and shield, and torchbearers trotted ahead and set fire to the wooden porticos along the street, lighting the way in the black gloom of the night. Then the Gothic trumpets blared, echoing across the sleeping City: *Beware! The Goths are upon you!* And with blood-chilling howls, the barbarian warriors charged down the long avenue into the maze of buildings and plazas of Rome.

More and more Goths entered the gate, an endless stream of barbarian warriors and war-horses. The bright avenue of flames stretched farther and farther into the distance. The summer had been dry; the flames caught readily, grew eagerly.

Finally, the last of the Gothic cavalry passed through the Salarian Gate and thudded down the street, echoing the distant, fading cry of Alaric's trumpets with their own. Now cries and screams of confusion and alarm were spreading throughout Rome as the citizens ran from their beds, hearing the howls and trumpets, now aware of the fires, aware that something was terribly amiss in the City.

Overhead, the sky was split by a brilliant streak of lightning and a roar of thunder.

The storm was upon the City.

Atawulf's sword slithered along iron and slashed into flesh, while overhead the clouds clashed in ear-splitting booms and eye-searing flashes. He spitted a City guardsman whose long lance he barely deflected with his shield. The fighting was fierce here, near the Capitol and forums and palaces, for by now resistance had converged, leaving the gates unguarded.

But there could never be enough resistance. Even now his younger brother Wallia should be at the Flaminian Gate, opening it to the barbarian foot soldiers—ten thousand warriors armed and waiting to come streaming into the most populated area of Rome.

The Bold Wolf slashed and stabbed viciously at the pitifully unprepared Roman soldiers, severing throats and limbs, riding the wounded down beneath Demon's hooves, the leather shoes now slippery with red.

His first sight of Rome was caught in flashing impressions of great buildings suddenly white-lit in the dancing glare of lightning, then just as suddenly gone; beautiful palaces catching fire, crowds of people fleeing, falling, their shrieks of terror swallowed up by the fury of thunderclaps overhead.

He drove his boot into a face, hacked at the neck as he passed; his shield caught a lance thrust, nearly unhorsing him, but his own swordthrust went home to the throat, and he rode on to slash deep through another's collarbone. On through the arcaded avenues he battled, seeing Rome through a spewing of red blood, a flickering of orange flames, a flaring of white lightning.

He kept Alaric ever in sight, the broad shoulders glinting with armor, and doggedly followed the huge white stallion along the maze of streets. A long wall loomed on one side, the red roofs of towering buildings intermittently visible in the flashing glare. The Goths wound beneath windows, arcades, balconies; Alaric led them ever upward, to higher ground, and Atawulf followed, leaving a bloody trail of bodies and limbs and entrails for the others to trample behind him.

Suddenly they were advancing up a slanting street, ascending one of the hills, losing men to a rain of arrows, but pressing forward with shields held high to protect themselves. They made the top of the street, meeting more resistance here than in the confusion and panic below. But not nearly enough lances and swords guarded that hill to halt the full onslaught of Gothic cavalry. Atawulf's Red Demon kicked and bit and plunged his way onto a large plaza overlooked by an imposing terrace and tiered balconies. There, under clashing and streaking skies, the crash and shriek of battle was as a silent shadow play on this insignificant hill, overpowered by the Olympic warring of the old gods in the roiling black clouds overhead.

Atawulf swung shield and sword ceaselessly, tirelessly, responding to a savage rhythm ancient to his blood, experience and instinct surer and quicker than thought, as he cut down one Roman after another. He took wounds, he knew, but none of them deadly, all of them forgotten in this contest of survival, blind slashing and thrusting until the few opponents left flung down their swords, dropped to their knees, and begged for mercy, begged to surrender.

Alaric accepted surrender and rounded up the Roman captives, placing them under guard. Now Atawulf felt the weariness in his limbs, but the fierce fire of battle still held him taut, still gleamed in his eyes. He swept his gaze over the City, a staccato scene under flashing skies, flames flickering here and there, and, from the direction they had come, a great fire glowing red off the clouds. He wiped the sweat from his face with the back of a bloody hand, turned his mount, and looked around to find the next assault.

Atawulf found no new assault. Between midnight and dawn the Goths had taken Rome and captured Palatine Hill.

Dia shot up from her sleep, sat up swiftly in bed; a crash of thunder so loud it seemed to shake the walls awakened her.

Then, between thunderclaps, there was something else. She heard the shouting of men, hobnail boots thudding on marble.

"Thalia, what is it?"

Thalia climbed upon the sleeping couch and huddled beside her. "I don't know, miss."

Dia's first thought was that the plebs had at last erupted into madness, that the mass of starving people were swarming up the Hill, making good their gruesome cry: *A price on human flesh!* She shuddered and clutched Thalia in the dark.

There was a commotion in the antechamber; her chamberlain came flying in, his face a mask of fear, frozen in a renewed flare of brilliant lightning, then gone again. She heard not a word he shrieked, so deafening was the roar of thunder. But in the next few flashes she saw armed men rush into the chamber. They were the City Guard, sent by the Prefect to hold her in custody in the House of Livia.

"Goths! . . . the City! . . . fighting . . . all over the Hill! Alaric . . . upon us! Flee!"

Unmindful of her thin chemise, Dia leaped from her bed, thinking to run and see for herself.

"Why aren't you defending the Hill?"

"Too late!" choked the head guardsman. "They're in the plaza!"

"They can't be on the Hill!" she cried in horror, but her words were swallowed up in another crack of thunder. Then Elpidia and Dulcie were there, slipping a thin mantle over her shoulders, and Thalia knelt before her with sandals; Dia sat down dazedly as her maid strapped them onto her feet.

They had her on her feet now, her maids and the nurse, urging her to flee. Were they truly fleeing the Goths in the midst of this wild storm? Surely this was a nightmare—surely she would awaken.

She looked around, irrationally, for her cat, but the old cat was nowhere to be found; in a storm like this she would be hiding under something, but before Dia could look under the dressing table she felt herself hurried from the room.

She stumbled between her determined rescuers in the vestibule, and lightning caught the bronze face on the bust of Livia. The Empress, in that swift series of flashes, regarded Placidia pityingly, admonishingly.

Dia resisted those who pulled her toward the door. "I shouldn't run; I should stay; Livia would stay."

The guard shook his head. Thalia tugged at her, terrified and pleading. Dia hesitated there in the vestibule. Every frantic pound of her heart, every trembling inch of her body screamed to her: *Run! Run! Hide!* Yet a small part of her resisted.

"Mother of God, what should I do?" She turned to her old nurse. "Pidi, what should I do?"

Elpidia took Dia's terrified face between her rough brown hands and looked at her young charge. The old nurse knew what an Imperial Princess should do; she should surround herself with guards and receive the Goths regally, trusting to her royalty to protect her. But was that possible with these savages? Was the reality of blood-crazed conquerors bursting upon them stronger and harsher than any royal claim she could make?

The matter was decided for them. There was the crash and clash of iron in the courtyard, heard as in a chaotic nightmare between the crash and clash of thunder. The guards, only a score, turned and raised weapons, and the women huddled behind them.

No polite delegation of soldiers came through the door, but a yelling, howling pack of blood-splattered barbarians. The Romans raised their weapons to meet the onslaught, but it was too much for Dia. She turned and fled, and all the women with her. They ran through the atrium and peristyle and dining room and into the outer garden, where the storm overhead only added to their panic.

Dia, who had lost her mantle during their flight, struggled frantically with the small barred door in the garden wall. She was crying in fear and helplessness as she sought desperately to open the door onto the narrow alley outside, praying and weeping unheard in the storm, her one thought escape from the demonic horde within the house.

At last the bar came free and they stumbled into the narrow passageway behind the House of Livia. Dia screamed as she tripped over the body of a slain guardsman and fell across another. Four others lay sprawled in the alley, cut down by passing barbarians.

Sobbing, she struggled to her feet. The women looked about wildly. There were several narrow passageways along which they could escape; there were steps descending Palatine Hill that would lead them into the streets, but what then? The streets would be more dangerous.

Suddenly a horseman appeared at the end of the passageway. The barbarian grinned horribly when he spied the women and urged his mount into the alley, followed by several others.

Too horrified even to scream, Dia and her maids and nurse scrambled back through the garden door and shoved it shut. Dia sobbed each breath as with trembling hands she struggled to drop the bar into the latch. Just as it fell into place, a heavy weight, like a man in armor, struck the door forcibly so that it rattled madly.

They backed away from the door. Between raging roars of thunder that seemed to rend the sky they heard iron on iron and screams in the palace and ugly laughter from the other side of the wall.

In a brilliant flare of lightning Dia saw the first grinning face rise over the wall. Then, in nightmarish motion, like a demon descending through a sea of light and dark, the man vaulted over the wall and dropped to the ground. Three more men appeared behind him, dropping swiftly into the garden.

Dulcie screamed and ran in panic, but Dia couldn't move. She stood frozen in terror even as Thalia tried to pull her away. But Elpidia placed herself between Dia and the Goth who advanced upon her, his ravenous eyes raking the curves beneath her thin chemise.

"Stop!" cried the nurse. "This is Imperial Prin——"

Shattering thunder took her words, and a huge hand slammed the old woman easily aside, knocking her to the ground.

Now Dia could move, but instead of running she shook Thalia off and started toward her fallen nurse. Rough, hard hands grasped her, pulled her back, and pushed her down onto the dry grass. Dia screamed and struggled, but the barbarian pressed her down easily with his huge thigh, laughing, his eyes a demonic yellow in the eerie light, his face ruthless with lustful joy.

She tried to fight, but he captured one hand and held it to the ground, and his armor was impervious to the feeble blows of her small fist. The Goth's free hand pawed her face, neck, and shoulder, cupped and squeezed her breasts through the thin linen of her gown. Then his head came down, his mouth forcing itself over hers, choking her cries, and he began to tug at the skirt of her chemise, pulling it higher, roving his rough hand over her bare thigh, and she felt she must die of shame and disgust and terror.

Suddenly the man above her grunted, as though the air were knocked out of him, and his crushing weight rolled aside. He came up swiftly, sword in hand, but the Goth who now stood over her held his own bloody sword ready, daring the other to attack.

"She's mine, Atawulf!" growled her attacker in rage.

"You're a fool, Sigeric!" the other snarled. "Such a fool I ought to cut you into little pieces, and that hairy lance you use for brains will be the first piece to go!"

Sigeric bellowed and flung himself at Atawulf, and as their swords clanged together Dia scrambled out from between them and crawled, shaking and crying, to Elpidia. The old woman folded the girl into her arms and rocked her as they huddled in the trampled flowerbed.

The other Goths halted to watch Sigeric and Atawulf fight, including the man who held Thalia struggling in his grip.

"I caught her," Sigeric gritted between clenched teeth as they locked swords. He threw his weight at Atawulf. "Find your own."

Atawulf shifted and flung Sigeric aside, caught the other's wild slash on his own sword, slashed rapidly in turn and drew blood across Sigeric's upper arm. Taking the other's furious return upon his shield, Atawulf in the same swift motion thrust inward. Sigeric leapt back to avoid the thrust. He glared at Atawulf, but held off; Atawulf was no man he wished to engage in a fight to the death; the Bold Wolf had personally escorted many a swordsman to the Gates of Hell.

Atawulf stood his ground, watching Sigeric. "If you think I'm out to steal your booty, then you're the biggest fool that ever rutted. Look around! Where the hell do you think you are?" Atawulf glared around at the men frozen in the garden like statues. "Not a man touches another woman on this hill!"

They glanced at each other. They had seen it coming; Atawulf had gone soft on them at last. The man who clutched Thalia by the arm let her go, and she stumbled numbly to join Dia and Elpidia.

"This is Palatine Hill, damn it! One of these women could be the Imperial Princess!"

The men shifted and eyed the women. Atawulf shouldered his shield, strode toward the huddled captives, and stared down at their trembling forms. Lightning danced upon the trio of women. His gaze fell on one beautiful, delicate face, framed in disheveled dark curls; startling translucent eyes stared up at him in wild fear.

Dia looked with horror into the savage face above her. Blood was smeared across his brow, nose, and cheek, gruesomely contrasting with dark blue eyes. The barbarian's beard, crimson-stained, had baubles braided into it, but the hair had fallen loose and hung tangled around the armored shoulders like some mangy lion's mane.

She shuddered, but she gathered her courage and did not turn away from those predatory eyes. Trembling, willing her knees not to buckle, she placed one hand on Thalia's shoulder and pushed to her feet, forced herself to stand, scarcely shoulder-height to this savage killer, and look into the grim, blood-streaked face that hovered over her.

She opened her mouth, tried to announce her identity, but thunder again shook the sky—fortunately, for no sound emerged from her terror-stricken throat beyond a small sob of fear. She dropped her eyes; she could not look at this nightmare of a man.

Atawulf saw that fear, the stark terror in the pale, oval face, the trembling chin and shoulders, but also recognized her struggle to overcome fear and stand unflinching before him. And those eyes! He wanted to see those strange eyes again.

He touched her, to lift her chin, and she jerked back in revulsion. His bloody thumb left a little smear of scarlet where he touched her chin.

He could not be sure of the color of those eyes in this dim, storm-obscured, early light, but he was sure of the revulsion he saw there. She set her jaw and lifted her head proudly, though she trembled all over, staring past him, unable to endure the sight of blood that had splattered him like rain. Nor could she endure that bold scrutiny which roved over her with no respect, no deference, only a predator's assessment of his prey.

Atawulf would have wagered a wagonload of gold that this tousled gem of a woman was the Imperial Princess, yet he must be sure. But before he could demand her identity, she drew herself up in a quiet lull in the storm and spoke with a quaking voice.

"I am Galla Placidia," she said as forcefully as she could manage through her trembling. Her only safety in this pack of brutes, she realized, was to make herself known to this one, who seemed to be the most ferocious, thereby a leader among these savages.

A white grin split the terrible, bloody beard. He never took his eyes from her, but his grating comment was directed to one of his men.

"Sigeric, if you had raped this one, Alaric would've personally carved you into wolfbait—slowly—starting with your balls."

Her attacker licked his lips determinedly. "She's still my captive."

Anger flashed in Atawulf's eyes. "She's the Emperor's sister. No greater hostage could we find in all the Empire. She belongs to Alaric. That's where I'm taking her, to keep her out of the greedy hands of more rutting fools."

Dia heard these words with relief, but she recoiled when the leader grasped her bare arm with his bloody fingers. As he started to pull her away, and the others closed in on Thalia, she cried out in protest.

"No! My maid! Leave her be!" The vehemence in her shriek gave him pause enough for her to continue. "She is my property; I forbid you to harm her. I require my maid and nurse with me or"—she faced the men imperiously—"or *Alaric* will hear of it, I assure you."

Atawulf burst out laughing. Despite the quaver in her voice, she had spoken in tones of royalty addressing her lessers, tones accustomed to obedience. And for a hostage to use the name of Alaric as a threat—well, it was too much.

She turned, astonished at his bellow of laughter. How could he laugh at the terror on Thalia's face? Tears sprang into her eyes as they met Atawulf's amused gaze, but she strove to face him down.

Atawulf felt the trembling of the small arm gripped in his fingers, and suddenly he was very glad he had saved her from the ravages of Sigeric, for he hated to imagine that tremulous brave face brutalized into submission. There was nothing Bold Wolf respected in man or woman more than courage, and this Roman princess was battling her fear with all the courage in her small frame.

He waved the men back with his reddened sword. "Bring your maid—and your nurse. Are there any more attendants you require, Your Royalty?"

He was still laughing at her, but he had acquiesced. "Thank you," she said carefully. "Only my maid Dulcie; that will be sufficient."

To her consternation, he burst out laughing again.

"Very well, Your Royalty. If we find this Dulcie, she is yours."

There was no need to find Dulcie. Upon hearing these words, she appeared from behind a box hedge where she had been hiding, scarcely daring to breathe. She crept forward, sidling around the armed men. Her pale face was streaked with dirt and tears.

Atawulf frowned at the buxom woman, the fair skin, the blond hair in disarray, the blue eyes.

"You cannot have this woman," he said.

Dulcie's blue eyes widened in renewed terror.

"Why not?" Dia insisted, no longer much afraid for herself since this barbarian had shown the sense to respect her rank, but afraid for Dulcie. "She's been my maid all my life. She's my property."

"She is not your property!" Atawulf snarled at her, suddenly finding her attitude offensive. "She is Germanni—one of us—and no longer slave to any Roman!"

Dia shook under the sudden fury of the Goth, the sudden tightening of the grip on her arm. She winced in real pain.

"Miss!" cried Dulcie. "Oh, miss, don't let them have me!"

"You're a free woman," Atawulf told her tightly. "Don't beg from her."

However flighty Dulcie seemed, she was no fool. And she had much experience of men, more than her mistress could ever imagine, and she had no illusions that being a free woman among the Gothic army would protect her from the warriors' lusts.

Dulcie stepped closer to Atawulf and gazed up at him timidly. "Am I free? Truly free?"

"Aye, woman. I have said it."

"Then I am most grateful. But Princess Placidia is . . . was . . . a kind mistress to me, and I would rest easier in my mind if you would allow me to accompany her to . . . to wherever you are taking her."

"You owe her nothing."

"No, I do not. But I know my . . . the princess was thinking only of my safety when she asked for me."

Atawulf's grip loosened as he regarded his royal captive. In his hesitation over Dulcie's request, Atawulf realized that the thunder and lightning had become less intense, and that the black clouds were now greying with the feeble dawn. A new sound invaded the garden, at first pattering and gentle, then of a sudden hissing and rattling as the wind picked up and a deluge of rain swept upon them.

"Inside." Without ceremony he dragged Dia across the garden and into the shelter of the house. By the time the women and warriors had gathered in the dining room they were dripping wet. Atawulf ordered his men to search the palace; the chamberlain was found and set to lighting the oil lamps on the elaborate gold stands.

Atawulf cursed to himself. He must keep the princess somewhere and search out Alaric in all this rain. Besides, there was much more to be done to secure the City. Dare he leave her here under guard?

He studied the delicate features, the fine nose and dainty chin, the curve of her full lips, those luminous eyes whose color wavered between blue and green in the fluttering light. Her hair was wet against her silky bare shoulders, and rested upon the rise and fall of those round breasts beneath the wet chemise, her rosy nipples enticingly visible beneath the thin white linen. If she were not the Imperial Princess, and if he were given to ravishing helpless captives . . .

But she was the Imperial Princess, the most valuable of their hostages. And he was *not* given to ravishing helpless captives. Atawulf knew captured cities. He had only to wait until business was finished; there would be plenty of *willing* women to choose from—perhaps even this Dulcie whose liquid blue eyes had gazed up at him so gratefully. But now another fact he knew of captured cities suddenly snapped him from his expectant musings.

"We've been here too long," he decided. "Sigeric, get your men together and mounted. There are other ripe hills to capture and rich houses to plunder—or would you have all the looters at your prizes first?"

Sigeric started to obey, then stopped and glared, looking from Atawulf to the princess suspiciously.

"She is for Alaric!" snapped Atawulf, his temper rising. "You'll find other women for the taking in those rich houses, if the rabble don't get to them before you. Go to it!"

With wordless resentment in the jut of his jaw, Sigeric signaled his men and tramped out of the dining room, leaving only Atawulf, a handful of his men, and the four captive women.

Atawulf realized he still gripped the princess's arm. He released her, and where his hand had been was a crimson stain of blood. She started to rub her arm, but jerked her fingers away in horror. Someone's life's blood was on her arm. She shuddered, suddenly feeling weak and sick. She groped for a chair, and Elpidia helped ease her into it.

I will not faint, Dia's thoughts tumbled. *I will not cry—oh, God, oh, God, what can I do? Blessed Mary, Blessed Virgin, save me from this nightmare—from these barbarians—from this horror of a man!*

She looked up at Atawulf, who still stood deep in indecision. Beneath the Roman armor and the red leather tunic there was nothing Roman about him. He was a powerful devil of destruction, taut and corded muscles gleaming in lamplight with a sheen of sweat, soot, and blood. Huge hands pushed back the mane of blood-plastered hair, and the thick blond brows lowered in concentration, the eyes of dark smoke-blue focused on his own thoughts. He looked no less wild, but she could see intelligence beneath the savagery, and that frightened her even more, as it would if wolves or boars should suddenly stand upright, speak, and conspire together against men.

Dia suddenly became uncomfortably aware of her state of undress. The wet chemise clung to her so revealingly, she might just as well be naked. She crossed her arms over her breasts, not realizing she presented an even more alluring picture to the barbarian.

Dia spoke in low tones to Dulcie, who, with an uneasy glance at the Goth, started from the dining room.

"Where are you going?" demanded Atawulf.

"To . . . to my mis——" Dulcie faltered. "I mean, I was just going to fetch the princess—"

"You'll go nowhere until I tell you."

Dulcie nodded and hurried back to her place beside her mistress's couch.

Dia swallowed her fear and gathered her nerve in a deep breath. "I only sent her for a mantle. Though I must insist you allow me to retire to my chamber and change into suitable clothes."

"No." Atawulf was letting none of them go anywhere without escort.

"No? You can't possibly expect me to receive Alaric in this state!"

It was well Bold Wolf had a keen sense of humor. *Receive Alaric?* The notion of his brawny brother in full armor presenting himself to her royal personage—as she seemed to expect—Alaric bowing and scraping like a courtier, why, the very idea made him snort with derisive mirth.

Dia was so affronted by his rude behavior that she forgot her modesty and dropped her hands into her lap, fists clenched.

Atawulf grinned at her. " 'Tis Alaric who will be receiving *you,* Your Uppityness—*King* Alaric, you'll have the courtesy to remember. And I think I would enjoy to distraction presenting you to my brother in that state."

"You wouldn't dare!"

The barbarian's dark blue gaze said quite plainly that he would dare. She suspected he was capable of subjecting her to any indignity; to avoid goading him, she decided she would be wisest to take a meeker approach. She twisted her fingers together nervously, not altogether sure how to go about being meek. But as she was genuinely terrified of what her fate might be, dragged before a conquering savage in naught but her chemise, there was real fear in her voice.

"As a royal hostage, I trust I may expect honorable treatment from . . . from a King of the Goths."

Then she abruptly looked up into the grisly red face of the savage and met the blue eyes squarely as the reference to his "brother" finally sank in. This marauding beast was brother to Alaric! The meekness was swiftly slipping from her voice as she spoke her mind on the matter of protocol, in which she was well schooled.

"Between noble houses there is always respect for royal hostages, even those at war. Your brother, the King, will not want to be party to any act which will demean his honor—or the honor of the Goths."

Atawulf's tawny brows dipped together as he considered her

words. She was right. He would be doing Alaric no favor if she was humiliated before Goths or Romans. She was the Imperial Princess, and Bold Wolf would not be the one to embarrass the King of the Goths by ill-treating her.

He shot a look at the princess. She was watching him expectantly, the nervousness gone from her demurely clasped hands and alert face. She knew beyond doubt, he thought, that she was right, and that he could do naught but concede it. He half-smiled; he had forgotten she was of that wily race—a Roman—and an Imperial at that. He would bear that in mind from now on.

Dia's confidence grew as she sat watching his face. He was considering her words. There was indeed intelligence there, more than just animal cunning, as she had first thought. The barbarian's expression told her he grasped the import to his brother's kingship—if leading a pack of dirty brigands and renegade slaves could be called such—and that he had no desire to jeopardize his brother's honor, whatever honor might consist of among the Goths.

When she saw the lips beneath the ghastly beard turn up wryly on one side, she relaxed somewhat and met it with an expression of royal affection learned from Serena and practiced to perfection in endless processions and ceremonies.

Her lips set into a curve that was not quite a smile, and Atawulf had the annoying feeling he was being condescended to. He scowled at her ferociously, but she did not shrink from his scowl, meeting it almost defiantly. Aye, she was an Imperial all right; he had almost forgotten that, taken in as he was by her girlish beauty, though he could all too clearly see she was no mere girl, but a shapely woman beneath that clinging, flimsy thing she wore.

The sound of pelting and hissing rain in the atrium brought him around to considering a course of action, any action, for contemplation of the lovely face and inviting curves of Princess Placidia was becoming a maddening distraction.

"All right, then," he snapped, angry at his own reaction. "Get yourself ready however you please. When Alaric settles into headquarters, I'll take you there. For now, I'll set a guard on you."

As he left abruptly to give orders to his men within the palace, Dia blinked in surprise. Whatever had made him snap like that at her? If anyone should be angry, she should be.

The enormity of her tragedy crashed in on her, now that he was gone. She was a prisoner of miserable savages. Rome was in their hands, and she was in their power. Soon that arrogant barbarian was going to parade her before Goths and Romans and hand her over to that brigand who called himself a king, making a mockery of royalty everywhere, and they would make a mockery of her. Who knew what Alaric was like?

The memory of Sigeric, that hulking brute, pressing his great weight down on her, running his hands over her breasts and thigh, smothering her with his disgusting, foul-smelling breath—she could not bear the horror and humiliation she felt.

Elpidia was babbling something at her, but she could only think of what happened in the garden—and, worse, what else surely would have happened if—no, she could not bear to think of it. As the shock following her terror and revulsion set in, Dia began to shudder, and soundless tears filled her eyes and spilled down her cheeks. She wished only to curl up in darkness; she wished to wake up and find this had all been a wretched, horrible nightmare.

Now violent sobs racked her body, and she turned to Pidi, dear, wise, comforting Pidi, and wept in her old nurse's embrace.

The Goths sacked Rome for three days, systematically looting the richest sections of the City and taking whatever plunder and women struck their fancy.

King Alaric ordered that there be no unprovoked killing and burning, but death and fires raged everywhere, for some of the slaves, seeing their chance at revenge in all the disorder, fell upon their masters and mistresses with the repressed fury of a lifetime.

The lawless elements among the plebeians, too, were just as vicious and destructive as the nobility always feared they would be if set loose. The City seethed with the turmoil of hatred and envy unchecked. Soon the people of Rome discovered they had more to fear from their fellow citizens than from the barbarian warriors.

The barbarians, at least, were under the control of one leader—a leader who had no interest in burning Rome to cinders or bathing her streets in blood. Alaric wanted her riches—all of them—and the savage joy of thumbing his nose at the Emperor by capturing and looting the prize of the Empire.

When Alaric stood in the shadow of the Arch of Titus, fists on narrow hips, mighty legs spread wide, the fire of victory in his massive breast, he saw carved upon the arch the triumphal procession of the Romans carrying the loot of Jerusalem before them out of that razed city. Alaric's handsome face broke into his dazzling wide grin.

He immediately set men to the task of finding among the gathered loot of the Capitol the trumpets and seven-branched candelabrum depicted on the triumphal arch. Rome's plunder would now be his. The prizes were found, and Alaric made a triumphal march of them along the Sacred Way, beneath the Arch of Titus, and up to the Great Palace.

Nothing was sacred to Alaric except the churches. The King of the Goths was Christian; the churches he ordered untouched, and he honored the right of sanctuary.

So it was a fine line of interpretation Sigeric trod when he set upon Marcella's house of Christian women.

Marcella's household was not literally a church, but a once-sumptuous estate on the Aventine. When Sigeric and his blood-stained men burst into the house, they expected exquisite furnishings and appointments, perhaps strongboxes of gold, silver, or jewels.

Instead they were received calmly by an old woman of eighty-five years and glowing eyes; she wore homespun, undyed wool, as did all the women within the household.

Sigeric demanded her gold. Marcella pointed out her coarse, unadorned tunic and declared she had no gold. She had given all her worldly goods for the succor of the poor.

Sigeric's men rounded up the dozen cringing, praying women, while some laid upon the aged Marcella with whips, determined to force her to reveal her hidden treasure. Marcella, however, flung herself at Sigeric's feet, pleading that they were all women of God. Tearfully she begged him to spare the younger women, among them her adopted daughter Principia, for they were virgins, dedicated Brides of Christ.

Sigeric cast the old woman aside. He and his men laid hands shamefully upon their trembling captives and tore at their garments.

Later it was said that Christ softened the barbarians' hearts and stayed their hands, but it was Alaric himself who, hearing the screams and prayers of the terrified women, entered the house and ascertained at once that they were what Marcella claimed them to be.

With curses that would have burned the holy women's ears if the words had not been in Gothic, Alaric ordered Sigeric to leave off harassing helpless females and find something profitable to do. Then Alaric sent the women to the Basilica of Saint Paul with an escort, and Marcella he sent carried in a litter.

Dia clung to the thin shoulders of her old nurse, and tears filled her eyes.

"Oh, Pidi, what will I do without you? How will I bear it?"

Elpidia's brown eyes danced with tears of her own. "You'll be fine, lovey. I know you will. You're my brave girl—only you're all grown up now, but I always thought I'd be with you, sweetling, dandling your babes on my knee . . ." The old woman sniffled, unable to go on.

"You will, Pidi. They can't keep me forever; I'll be back as soon as Honor settles with them. Oh, what am I crying for? I always wanted out of this musty old palace."

"I'm going to give that Atawulf a piece of my mind—saying I'm too old for a trip like this. I've traveled in wagons and coaches since I was knee-high, and when I went east with Empress Justina, there we were with your mother and Justa and Grata and little Val—three young princesses and a boy barely old enough to toddle, much less be Emperor, poor thing—running for our lives after the old Emperor died—"

Dia, having heard this tale a thousand times and suddenly realizing that Elpidia must be quite old by now—in her sixties, at least—pulled back and smiled at her nurse through tear-blurred eyes.

"You'd travel with the best of them, I'll bet. But, Pidi, he's made up his mind, and arrangements are made; it's too late to change them now . . ." Her voice caught at the thought of what might lie ahead, for Atawulf was waiting to escort her to the City gates even now. Dia forced herself to go brightly on, so as not to distress the old woman further.

"Besides, who'll take care of this crotchety old cat while I'm gone? And what an adventure this will be! Aunties Justa and Grata will be green with envy when they hear of it!"

Dia could not go on, for she did not believe a word of her bright prattle. She was going off with an army of savages.

She squeezed her nurse's weathered brown face between her hands. "Good-bye, Pidi, darling. I'll miss you terribly, but I *will* come home; I promise."

It occurred to Dia then that Elpidia was so old, that if she were gone a very long time her nurse might not still be living when she returned. She thrust that chilling thought aside and kissed the withered lips.

"Good-bye, baby," whispered Elpidia, clinging to her child, the sun of her life. "I'll be here waiting to welcome you home— that's my promise. Now, don't you let that Dulcie get too saucy."

"I won't," Dia half-laughed through her tears. "I love you, Pidi—do you know that?"

"I know it, honey. And I don't have to tell you—" The old woman nearly broke down.

"No, you don't." Dia hugged Elpidia one last time, then turned and fled the vestibule so blindly that she ran straight into Atawulf. Startled, Atawulf caught at her, but she skirted around him, eyes blinking. The two handmaidens awaited Dia in the courtyard—Thalia pale and anxious, Dulcie flushed and excited.

Dia turned back for one last look at the House of Livia, her home for so many years. Elpidia stood in the doorway, forlornly watching her departure. With a painful lump in her throat, Dia waved and turned quickly away. In the avenue outside the courtyard stood an Imperial carriage, with four beautiful white mares waiting patiently, flicking their tails at flies.

Dia and her maids seated themselves in the plush purple-and-gold appointed carriage which would convey them southward through the City to the Appian Gate. Alaric wished the Imperial Princess to be on view to the populace—his prize, his triumph—and as the carriage moved down the slope of the Palatine, Dia saw that the people had turned out to watch the Goths' departure—and her abduction.

Her carriage joined the procession of Goths leaving the City, a train of wagons laden with loot, with Dia displayed in the van like prize plunder. She burned with humiliation. Escorted by a hundred Gothic horsemen, the golden carriage moved through the warm, clear morning, winding its way through the streets of Rome between rows of the citizenry gathered to watch the Goths depart.

I'm like Helen, dragged from Troy by the Greeks—or Zenobia, paraded through Palmyra by Emperor Aurelian.

I am Galla Placidia. I will not show fear or shame or tears—I cannot!

Dia held her head high and looked neither right nor left, as befitted a princess of the royal house, and strove to maintain an expression of serene dignity, as though this were any other royal procession, as though the daughter of Theodosius were above the petty actions of a lot of marauding barbarians.

The people, she realized as she glanced surreptitiously out the open window, fell silent as her carriage passed. Most of the faces were sober, grave, and shadowed with sorrow, for this was a momentous defeat for Rome, they knew—this taking hostage of the Imperial Princess—and who knew what portent of the future?

Here and there drunken revelers hailed the carriage with whistles and catcalls, but Atawulf sent horsemen charging among them. The princess was meeting this bravely, and he had seen her quick intake of breath when the plebeian scum jeered. He did not want any mishap to break down her courage.

Dia did not know whether to feel relieved or heartbroken when they at last reached the Appian Gate. Outside the walls, she and her maids alighted from the carriage. She accepted Atawulf's hand, trembling. The entire Gothic nation gradually assembled outside the walls, ready to move on, richer by hundreds of wagons laden with the spoils of Rome.

Atawulf escorted her to a royal sleeping coach drawn by eight strong mules—the coach which would be her home among the landless Goths.

Bold Wolf's blue eyes were grave, but his voice teased. "I hope, Your Royalty, your quarters are not too primitive or barbaric."

"I told you—the Imperial women are a hardy breed. We travel as well as any Goth."

Atawulf grinned. "We'll see, Princess."

Before she entered the sleeping coach, Princess Placidia took one last look at the walls of Rome and the Appian Gate. Red roofs glowed in the morning sunlight, warmly inviting her back into the familiar streets, buildings, and forums. Tears blurred her vision.

"Come, dears," she said softly to her maids, "we'll think of it as a grand adventure. Such tales we'll have for the aunties."

4

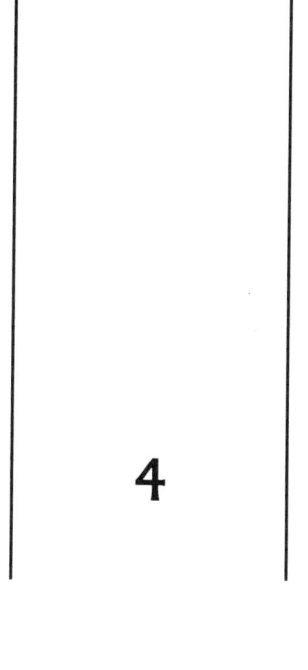

LORD, IT was hot.

Dia waved the ivory-and-silk fan listlessly, stirring oven-baked air without raising even an illusion of a breeze.

She had long ago given up on relieving the oppressive heat. Dulcie still wrestled with her own fan vigorously, but Thalia no longer bothered, leaning wearily against the side of the stuffy coach.

Stuffy even with all the windows flung open and the curtains tied back. Who could say which was worse—leaving the curtains open to the scorching sun which beat mercilessly into the coach, or drawing the curtains and blocking the little breeze that might find its way from the sea?

Already Dia had lost count of the days they traveled with the Goths. Was it a week? A fortnight? It seemed longer.

A lifetime ago, it seemed, the gates of Rome dwindled behind her, tall cypress shading the silent and somber tombs along the Appian Way.

The Goths had traveled swiftly at first, at dusk erecting tents and pulling them down before first light; eating cold gruel, hard bread and cheese, salt-dried meat, washing it down with sour vinegar wine. But the farther south the army caravan traveled, the more fresh mutton, mullet, geese, and cabbages appeared. Dia thought fleetingly about where the food came from. They stole the food, she imagined, from farms and estates that had managed to hide their stores from other raids.

Worse than the rough, monotonous fare, though, was the scarcity of water. The south of Italia was suffering from drought, and water was as much sought by scouts as was food. Oh, Alaric made sure his royal hostage had plenty of drinking water—it would not do to have her wasting away from thirst—but bathing water was absolutely forbidden.

Dia could scarcely remember a time in her life when she did not bathe leisurely and languorously every day. Summer and winter she dipped in the hot, warm, and cold baths of the palace. In winter she lingered in the steam rooms; in summer she swam in the outdoor pools.

Alaric would not allow her enough water even for a sponge bath. If the horses and people were thirsty, he saw no reason why the princess should be indulged—as if washing her hair were an indulgence!

Dia would have fretted and fumed if the heat had not drained all the energy from her. She smelled as bad as a barbarian. She could scarcely stand her own company or bear her own skin.

Now, as the Appian Way neared the seacoast, she found the closeness of the coach unbearable. When she knelt on the cushions and put her face to the window, catching the slight sea breeze, she could smell the fresh salt air, and her longing to be out under the open sky was overpowering.

None of the three women had spoken a word for miles, all possible complaints and lamentations of the heat long since exhausted, expressed now only in occasional heavy sighs and renewed exertions of their fans. Therefore, when Dulcie spoke, her sudden exclamation startled the other two.

"Oh, miss, here he comes again!"

Dulcie turned from where she had been staring out the window and smiled.

"He's come to ask after your health again, Miss Dia."

"Let's tell him I've died."

"Since he last checked an hour ago?"

"Tell him to fling my body into the sea, where at least in death I'll be clean and cool."

"He comes just to see you, you know."

"Nonsense! He comes because he's terrified I'll die of heat prostration and filth." Dia flung herself on her back across the cushions and folded her hands over her bosom, assuming a funereal pose.

The clip-clop of the red stallion's hooves upon the pavement was barely discernible amid the constant clatter of coach wheels and mules' hooves. From the horse's back, Atawulf leaned forward and peered into the coach.

"Still in a sulk, Your Royalty?"

"Princess Placidia has died," Dulcie told him flatly.

"Eh?" Atawulf stared at her as if he hadn't heard aright.

"Her last request was that you fling her body into the sea."

"*What?*" roared Bold Wolf, glaring into the coach. He could just make out the form of the princess lying serenely on her back, hands folded. His first thought was that the little fool had somehow managed to kill herself. Or perhaps she truly had succumbed to the heat. She had barely answered his solicitous questions an hour ago, and then she had told him sharply to go away and leave her to suffer in peace.

Swearing in Gothic, Atawulf wrenched open the side door of the coach and dropped his solid weight into the conveyance. The coach rocked. Before Dia could move she felt her arms grasped in iron fingers, which jerked her up and shook her roughly.

"Princess!" Bold Wolf thrust his face into hers in the dim light and searched for a reaction.

He got one.

"Aayyhh! Let go of me, you beast! How dare you lay hands on my person!"

"How dare I! Your maid said—"

"Obviously she was joking!" Dia snapped, futilely trying to wrench free of his strong grip. Why, the man was half-naked, his broad bronze shoulders bare and close and radiating the heat of the noonday sun.

His grip tightened. "Obviously. What kind of trick are you up to?"

"Trick?"

"I'm not a fool. Did you think to invent some ruse to escape?" He shook her again, furious at the panic that had raced through him.

"Stop it! Stop shaking me!"

"Answer me!"

To his dismay she began to cry in great, heaving sobs. He abruptly released her bare arms, and she immediately buried her face in them. Her shoulders shook with muffled, choking convulsions.

Atawulf was instantly contrite. "I shouldn't blame you for trying to escape, Princess. 'Tis no more than a woman of the Goths would do in your place."

His broad hand went out to her. When he touched her hair, Dia flung her head back and looked full into his eyes. Hers were dancing with tears—tears of mirth. Great peals of laughter shook her bare shoulders.

"You should have seen your face!" she gasped with delight. "You were horrified, weren't you? I could just see you wondering how to tell Alaric his precious hostage was dead! Oh, priceless!"

Atawulf's concerned expression stiffened. "What makes you think a stupid ruse like that could fool me for more than an instant? For an escape plan it was damned—"

"Escape?" Dia laughed sharply. "It was a joke, just a joke. Whoever thought you would fall for it?"

"A joke!" Atawulf shook her sharply by the shoulders. "You find it amusing to laugh at me?"

"Why not?" Suddenly she was angry, childishly, petulantly angry. "You laughed when I was nearly . . . nearly . . . when I was captured—and even when I humbled myself and asked to see Alaric."

Abruptly she pulled out of his grasp. *"Now* where's your sense of humor, Atawulf? Not so funny when the great Gothic warrior is the butt of the joke?"

Atawulf stared at the Imperial Princess with disbelief hanging slack on his face. Then he grinned, the grin grew into a deep-chested chuckle; finally he dropped his head back and rocked the coach with huge guffaws.

While Dulcie giggled and Thalia stared wide-eyed, Dia glared, genuinely piqued that the man did indeed have a sense of humor.

Atawulf shook his head. "I didn't know you had it in you, Your Royalty! You've gotten over your sulks, have you, and begun enjoying yourself?"

"No! I am *not* enjoying myself. I'm miserable!" she snapped at him. "I'm cooped up in this miserable coach where it's hot and sweltering and I can't get any breeze at all. There's nothing to do all day and it's so boring I can't bear it."

" 'Twas yourself, I believe, who insisted on traveling in luxury."

"This is not luxury! I'm sticky and filthy and I'm not even allowed the simple courtesy of a *bath!*"

"Bath? Water is in short supply—nobody gets a bath."

"You Goths are used to it, no doubt. I am not."

Atawulf glared, annoyed by the imperious lift of her chin. "Well, Your Snootiness," he drawled harshly, "perhaps you Romans just naturally *stink* more than we Goths." Savagely he kicked at the coach door and whistled for his horse.

"No! Wait!" As he was about to leap upon the red stallion's back, Dia swallowed her pride, the taste bitter in her mouth. *"Please!"*

Atawulf checked his leap and turned around, his face a mask of disbelief.

"Please?" He stuck a little finger in one ear and made a great show of clearing the passage out. "I seem to be hearing things. Did you say—*please?*"

"I did. You needn't be sarcastic."

"And you needn't be a pain in the ass."

"Well, I never heard such insensitive— *I* am not the one who dragged *you* against your will on this endless journey in this wretched heat."

"If I remember correctly, it was *you* who claimed the Imperial women were a hardy lot, and that I'd hear no complaints."

Dia glared at him. True, she had said that, but it galled her to have it thrown in her face. She answered with a regal toss of her head.

"I've changed my mind. The heat in this coach is intolerable. I de—— I mean, I would like you to make other arrangements."

"These were the arrangements you wanted, Your Royalty."

"I know that," she said crossly. "Stop flinging my words back at me. What do you want me to say? I was wrong? All right—I was wrong! Are you satisfied?"

Atawulf grinned broadly. "Tolerably. Just what do you expect me to do about the heat, Princess? Everyone's suffering, the same as you."

"Everyone isn't shut up in this stuffy old thing. You certainly aren't; you ride about as you please in the open air, at least. I . . . *request* the privilege of the same."

"You *ride?*" he drawled.

Dia ignored his sarcasm.

"Of course I ride. I ride superbly."

"Naturally."

"You don't believe me?"

"Oh, I believe you, Princess. I'm looking forward to seeing you ride a war-horse. Why not start with mine? Red Demon."

"Your constant mockery is becoming quite tiresome. Good day." She turned her head away dismissively.

He clucked his tongue. "What a sharp temper you have, Miss Imperial. Now where is *your* sense of humor?"

Dia allowed herself a small smile of triumph while her face was still turned away. Since Atawulf had not departed right away, he must truly intend to let her ride. These Goths! They simply would do nothing without first indulging in a good argument.

She turned to face him with a look of exasperation. "Lord Atawulf, or whatever your people call you . . ."

"Atawulf. I need no *Roman* title."

"Very well, Atawulf . . . I'm sure you know I've never ridden a war-horse, nor do I intend to. I'm equally sure you can find me a suitable mount. Naturally it must be a mount suited to royalty . . ."

"Naturally."

"Perhaps a dainty little mare, not too gentle, not too jumpy. Then we can continue this fascinating verbal contest in the saddle."

Atawulf's blue eyes narrowed. "Princess, you are the most arrogant woman I've had the misfortune to meet. What makes you think I have the time or the inclination to cater to your royal whims?"

Her sulky lips curved up in a sharp smile. "I'm certain you're curious as to whether I'll make a fool of myself."

His dark blue eyes sparkled. "I'll admit I find the idea tempting. All right, but don't complain if your royal butt gets saddle sore."

When Atawulf had gone to find her a horse, Dia fell back against the cushions. "Well, I never— the nerve of that man."

"Oh, he's a bold one, miss," laughed Dulcie, "as a man should be. And handsome, too, you'll admit."

"I'll admit no such thing. He's barbaric! That awful beard! And he might put on a tunic instead of going naked on top like a . . . a wrestler. Furthermore, I've never been so rudely spoken to in my—"

"But he *is* taking you riding, miss." Dulcie sighed. "I wish it was me."

Dia sat up abruptly. "I must be ready. Dulcie, find me a clean dress for riding, something cool. Thalia, quick, rebraid my hair, string some jewels in it. And you can stop smirking, both of you. I'm not trying to impress that arrogant barbarian. If I'm going to be stared at by the whole Gothic nation, they're going to see that the Imperial Princess is a *royal* hostage and not to be cowed by a lot of ragtag vagabonds."

By the time Atawulf returned, Dia was dressed in a summer dress of palest blue linen shot through with silver threads. The light garment was sleeveless, and Thalia girded it at Dia's waist with a belt of silver rope, letting the soft material blouse over breezily. She girded it with another belt low on the hips, again blousing the material loosely, so that the chemise's fullness was pulled up short enough for riding—her hem falling just below the knees.

Beneath the loose folds of the thin material Dia wore a narrow cloth band to keep her breasts from jouncing immodestly, and beneath the skirt she wore a soft linen undergarment which hugged her thighs—a gentlewoman's version of the short hunting pants noblemen sported.

As Atawulf bid the driver to halt the slow-moving coach, he was met with a vision of girlish loveliness framed in the gilded doorway. Bare arms and shoulders of silken smoothness. Bare calves, slim and shapely—of which he wisely said nothing, not wishing to arouse any sudden modesty in the nymph poised before him—delicate ankles encircled with the narrow straps of her silvery sandals.

Suddenly gallant, the Bold Wolf leapt from Demon's back and caught the tiny waist in the huge span of his hands, lifting the startled princess easily down to the pavement.

She shoved his hands away hastily. "I am perfectly capable of descending on my own, thank you."

"You're welcome," he said dryly.

But her attention was now on the white mare he had on lead. "Oh, my, she's a beauty."

"She ought to be. She's from the Imperial stables."

"Naturally."

He linked his brawny fingers together. "A hand up, Princess? Or is mounting something you are perfectly capable of doing for yourself?"

She considered refusing his help, but springing from the ground into the saddle was a difficult feat. She might not make it on the first try, and she was determined not to give this overbearing barbarian the slightest excuse to laugh at her attempt.

"A hand up, please," she said, trying so hard to assert her dignity she managed to make even the "please" sound imperious. She lifted a dainty sandaled foot into his hands and grasped the saddle. Abruptly she was flying over it, as the barbarian launched her into the air much more energetically than was necessary. Grabbing frantically at the saddle, she barely managed to keep from tumbling off the other side. The mare danced skittishly, but Dia kept her seat.

Dia glared down at the delighted Goth as she righted herself. Then, to her displeasure, he turned and easily vaulted onto the huge war-horse. She took up her reins and pretended not to notice.

The coach had lurched into motion while they mounted, lumbering along with the caravan. As their two horses came abreast of the coach, Dulcie put her head out a window.

"Oh, Miss Dia, beg pardon, but 'tis terrible hot in here for us, too. Could we be allowed to ride up top, Thalia and me?"

"Of course you may," answered Dia. She deliberately did not glance Atawulf's way. She, after all, was in charge of her own women, not he. Her tone dared him to interfere. "Driver, stop the coach and make room for my maids."

The driver, a muscular, barrel-chested man with a drooping

mustache and limp topknot, looked to Atawulf for orders. Atawulf nodded assent, his face expressionless, but his blue eyes brimmed with amusement. Eagerly, the driver halted the mules; he certainly had no objection to female company on a long day's ride.

Dia did not miss the fact that the driver stopped at Atawulf's order, not hers, but she was just glad for small blessings; Atawulf had not countermanded her order, but let it stand. Perhaps this would be a pleasant ride after all.

The maids clambered onto the coach top, Dulcie happily taking a seat beside the driver, while Thalia timidly settled cross-legged upon the roof behind them. The Greek slave was still wary of the barbarians, and she had been unusually quiet ever since the beginning of this journey. Still, she was so grateful to be out of that oven of a coach that a happy smile lit her narrow face.

"Thank you, Miss Dia," she said shyly, wishing she could be as bold and saucy as Dulcie; but then, Dulcie was a free woman now, and Thalia was not.

Atawulf pressed his knees to Demon's sides and led the way off the highway. The Appian Way, twenty-four feet wide and paved with flat stones, the smoothest and swiftest route along the uneven coastline, was crowded with hundreds of wagons and carts pulled by mules and oxen—wagons and carts in which the Goths carried children and tents, household goods, armor, and most of the movable finery of Rome.

Atawulf's mount led the way across the wide, shallow drainage ditch to the left of the highway and onto fairly flat ground, weedy with brown grass and wilted scrub brush. The horses' hooves sent lizards scurrying and rustling through the brittle underbrush. Here, threading among clusters of juniper, bramble, broom, and laurel, the caravan was less crowded, but men—and a few women—on horseback stirred up dust as they tramped along, dust which added one more misery to the vagabonds on foot, those with no horse or wagon, who by the end of the day would struggle into camp weary and dust-caked.

Atawulf reined in the war-horse to let the white mare step up beside him.

"Miss Dia?" he drawled teasingly. "So you do have a name besides Her Royal Snootiness."

"I am addressed as Most Noble Imperial Princess Galla Placidia."

"Aye, a name as heavy as that purple cloak you packed along, and about as useful. You won't mind if I call you Dia?"

"I *do* mind."

"Dia suits you better. A childhood nickname, is it?"

"Only the closest members of my household may call me by that name. Certainly not a Count of the Domestic Horse, which you profess to be."

"You may call me Bold Wolf," he offered teasingly.

"I will not. It sounds vulgar and . . . brutish." She cut her eyes at him measuredly. "Though perhaps it suits you."

"Meaning?"

"Meaning you couldn't drag a pitchfork through that shaggy hair, and you might shave that wretched beard. What did you cut it with—a saw?"

"Oh, I don't look enough the gentleman to be in your sacred presence?"

"A gentleman you will never be."

Atawulf grinned at her. "Now we're getting somewhere. Thanks."

"That was not a compliment."

"Oh, aye, it was. There's not a Gothic warrior alive—or dead—who wants to be called a gentleman."

"I can well believe that."

Atawulf's grin broadened as his gaze followed the smooth curve of her bare neck and shoulder and slid along the silky line of her slender arm. Her narrow wrist was relaxed as she held the reins loosely in her fingers. Then his eyes dropped to the rounded knee and shapely leg hugging the horse, gracefully outlined against the mare's whiteness in the stark sunlight.

"I'm pleased to confess I find your appearance easier on the eyes than you do mine. I wouldn't change a thing, except maybe I'd put a smile on those pouty lips."

"You are determined to annoy me, aren't you?"

"You're the one who invited herself riding—remember? I'm just as set on enjoying the ride as you are on being miserable."

She looked at him sharply. "You think I like being miserable?"

"You revel in it."

"Oh, you!"

"But it won't work. Everything I say throws that snooty little nose into the air, but you know something? I love it." Atawulf's tone was taunting. "I'm going to do you a favor and give you every excuse to be just as miserable as you want to be."

Dia turned in the saddle, rounding on him furiously. "I do *not* appreciate your high-handed attitude or your sarcasm. You don't know anything about what I want."

"Then tell me."

"I want my freedom!"

He shook his head. "That I can't give you."

"Won't," she corrected.

"All right—won't. Anything else?"

She sighed. "No. Yes, I . . . never mind." She had been about to say she wanted a bath, but she knew such a request would elicit more sarcasm and insult from the Goth. Sweat and dirt were a second skin to him, she thought. Then ruefully it occurred to her they were becoming a second skin to her, too. She wondered if she smelled as awful as she felt.

She rode in silence, determined to ignore him, looking about the parched bushland as though its dry stillness held endless fascination. The horses' hooves thudded loudly on baked earth, a comforting familiar rhythm broken only occasionally by the brittle rustle of swallows taking wing at their approach, or sundered by the raucous cries of ravens. And always the background clop and clatter, rattle and rumble of thousands of heavy hooves and wooden wheels on paved stone, a nation on the move.

A nation going nowhere. A people without a home.

Dia's gaze fixed upon the Gothic warrior riding ahead of her, his hair the color of harvest-heavy wheat, his broad shoulders bare and sun-bronzed. The hard terrain of his muscled arms, ringed with bands of gold and garnet, brought to her mind the contained heat of a volcano—explosive power beneath the contoured surface. His back rippled with rugged force as he moved his body to the rhythm of the horse beneath him. Strong, leather-clad thighs gripped the stallion, tireless, as though he had been born to merge his strength with his mount, fashioned by nature to spend a lifetime on horseback.

He was the quintessential picture of the savage barbarian warrior, full of power and virility.

Dia could just hear what Aunt Grata would say if she were here now. *My, how that man does sit a horse.*

Shocked at the wanton wanderings of her own mind, Dia drew her thoughts in sharply and, inadvertently, the reins of her mount. The little mare danced sideways and jerked her head in vigorous protest.

Atawulf circled his horse and looked back to see if something was amiss, and Dia, to her horror, felt a heated flush rising to redden her cheeks. Fearing he might read her thoughts in her heightened color, she bent her neck and brushed at the beaded perspiration on her forehead.

"It's this heat," she said breathlessly. "I should have brought a fan."

Atawulf steered the stallion to her side, concerned. "You're red as a cherry tart."

"I beg your—"

"We've got to cool you down—*now.*" Atawulf had seen

strong men turn this red in the heat—and die of it. Hurriedly he unstrung the waterskin from his saddle, uncorked it, and shoved it in her face.

"Drink," he ordered. "Just a few swallows."

Since she was thirsty, she complied, tipping her head back and letting the liquid stream into her mouth. As she drank, her eyes cut sidewise to Atawulf. Worry furrowed his brow, and the intense anxiety in the stormy blue eyes gave her pause. He truly believed she was overcome with the heat; he would panic indeed if she should faint from her horse.

The thought made her laugh, and suddenly she was choking on the water, gasping and coughing.

"Enough," he said, taking the waterskin from her. "You shouldn't drink too much. Best to cool down from the outside." He poured water into his palm and gingerly stroked his broad hand across the delicate curve of her neck where stray locks of hair lay loose and damp.

Dia jerked in surprise, but the cool wetness was soothing and felt wonderful on her hot skin.

Atawulf filled his hand again and dabbled more water over the nape of her neck, spread it with his palm gently across her back and shoulders, and to him her skin felt like warm satin, soft, with a rich, radiant glow.

Dia blushed even more furiously. She sidled her horse out of his reach.

"I'm all right now . . . really. You needn't . . ." Drawing on her dignity, she faced him. "Thank you for . . . your concern, but I think we should ride on now."

"No, we shouldn't." He caught at the mare's bridle and dismounted from his own horse. He opened his strong hands, ready to assist her. "If you haven't recovered fully, riding on could be deadly. Come on. We're going to sit down."

Dia looked down at his serious face in resignation. Short of admitting that she had never felt faint with heat in the first place, she would never convince him she felt fine. But she wanted so badly to ride free on this brilliant, hot day, and she was thoroughly sick of submitting her wishes to those of senators, royal guards, and barbarians.

Rebelliously, she kicked her mare into a lunge, free of the grasping fingers of the startled barbarian, and pressed the little horse into a canter. The clustered trees and brush slowed the mare until she emerged upon a grassy knoll and followed a low ridge upward.

She urged the white mare to quicken her pace on her headlong gallop uphill. Dia rode low to the white-maned neck and did not risk a backward glance until they topped a promontory dotted with cluster pines. From the top of the hill she could see the sea, an expanse of sparkling blue, brilliant in the sun. A whisper of sea breeze carried a whiff of salt water. In the instant she paused, breathing the tangy air, she turned and looked down the hill.

Atawulf had remounted, and Red Demon now covered the ground between them at a breakneck pace. The Gothic warrior's lips curled back in a dangerous snarl.

If Dia entertained any notion of waiting for him, the fury in his face quelled it. Then she spied the path plunging toward the seashore. She urged her mount down the path at reckless speed.

Between the hillock and the sea, however, lay the Appian Way and the Gothic caravan. Dia raced her mare alongside it and slipped through a gap between wagons just under the noses of two oxen who did not even blink at her sudden passage. Nor did they blink at Atawulf's abrupt breakthrough just moments later.

Jeers and catcalls burned Atawulf's ears as he sped after the fleet mare.

"Let her get away already, eh, Bold Wolf?"

"What'd you do—kiss her?"

Atawulf snarled over his shoulder.

Onto the beach the mare galloped, spraying sand in rapid staccato beneath her hooves. Dia pushed her onward, leaning forward, gripping with her knees and urging the horse with sweet words. They raced parallel to the waterline, then closer, raising a fine spray as the white mare splattered the water.

Dia laughed aloud, startling herself, for she had not laughed from sheer pleasure since . . . why, since she signed the order for Serena's execution. She looked back; Atawulf was gaining on her, the muscular legs of his great red war-horse pounding the distance between them into nothing.

"Go, girl," she encouraged the mare. The white horse leapt over driftwood, long mane and tail flying, and far ahead Dia spied the thatched roofs and smoke of a fishing village. For the first time the idea of escape, real escape, entered her mind, and she thought wildly of galloping into town for protection—there would be a church, and even Alaric respected the Church's right of sanctuary.

"*Go!*" she cried, and she almost sobbed her urgency, but at that moment sinews of iron encircled her, and she was plucked roughly and ignominiously from her mount.

She cried out, beating at the massive forearm around her waist, kicking the air ineffectually in an effort to wrest free. Atawulf reined in his mount; the white mare pounded down the beach a short distance, until she realized she had lost her rider, and, snorting, slowed to a standstill.

Dia twisted around and glared up into a face of rage. Perhaps struggling was not the wisest course. She forced herself to be still and sat stiffly upon his thigh. Trying to retain an air of dignity, she stared stonily down the beach. Her horse stood staring at them, ears pricked forward, waiting to see what might happen next.

"You little bitch!" Atawulf hissed between drawn lips.

"I've given you no cause to call me rude names."

"Haven't you? No, I guess you've just been doing what comes naturally to a Roman. Like a fool, I swallowed every lie and every trick."

"I'm sure I don't know what you're talking about."

His arm tightened abruptly, and she gasped for breath. Never loosening his hold about her waist, he swung one leg over the saddle and dropped them both to their feet in the sand. His fingers dug into her bare arms as he held her facing him.

"All that pleading to go riding, and then pretending to be overcome with the heat—all tricks to gain my sympathy, lies to catch me off-guard so that you could escape. Well, it nearly worked, Miss Imperial Majesty, but it never will again."

Dia stared at him in astonishment. Why, the man believed every word he spoke, and had worked himself into a froth of anger over a series of unconnected events. She felt like laughing.

"That's ridiculous," she sputtered. "You can't possibly imagine—"

"I don't have to imagine!" He shook her roughly. "But it was a stupid idea. All you accomplished was to make a fool of me, but that won't happen again either."

Dia's eyes widened in sudden comprehension, then narrowed into feline slits. She had pricked his pride. *Well, what of my own pride?* she fumed to herself. She was not about to tell him his suppositions were wrong, to grovel and plead innocence, especially admit that what he had taken for feigned sunstroke was embarrassment at the indecency of her own wayward imagination. *If his pride is that fragile, let it beware!*

"Naturally, I tried to escape," she told him frostily. "If you were the one held captive, it's the first thing you would do, too. If I had to trick you to escape"—she shrugged—"how foolish you feel about it is your problem, not mine."

But the Bold Wolf's pride was not that fragile. His deep-set blue eyes bored into hers. Her carefully coiled braids had half fallen, along with the loops of jewels, and wispy strands of deep brown hair trailed over her flushed cheeks and caressed her slim neck. Her silky skin blazed, her color heightened to a vibrant glow with exertion and emotion.

She raised her eyes and met his boldly.

Atawulf dropped his hands and paced away from her. Then he spun about in the sand to stare at her for another long moment.

He shook his shaggy head, and a slow grin crept across his features.

"Aye," he drawled. "If I were captive, I'd do the same. I'd use every opportunity at hand to escape. Being female, you use trickery a man would not."

"Oh, you would if you had to, Atawulf. Only you'd call it cleverness, being male."

He laughed, a sharp bark of merriment.

"Princess, I vow, you did as well as any woman of the Goths."

"No," Dia countered, "I did as well as any woman of the Romans."

Atawulf scowled. " 'Twas a compliment. Do not insult our women."

"Do not insult ours. I am pure Roman. Any virtues I possess are pure Roman, and I am as proud of that as any woman of the Goths is proud of her own."

"Aye, you're pure Roman all right—and an Imperial. I'm not likely to forget."

"I won't let you forget."

"I've no doubt of that." He caught the reins of his Red Demon. "Let's call a truce, Your Royalty, at least long enough to ride back in an agreeable fashion."

"I'm willing."

Atawulf mounted and rode after the white mare. He handed the reins over to Dia. When he showed no signs of dismounting and helping her up, she gripped the saddle, gritted her teeth in determination, and leapt, managing to fling one leg over the horse's rump. Inelegantly, she hoisted herself into the saddle.

Watching her, Bold Wolf was rewarded with a glimpse of shapely knee and thigh and undergarment. Dia, noticing his gaze, pulled the hem of her girded-up dress a little lower, covering her knees. She shifted uncomfortably on the hard leather saddle and had reason to be glad of the short linen leggings worn by noblewomen when riding. She was accustomed to a softer seat than the rough red leather, which chafed in the most delicate places. Her own favorite saddle had been sensibly lined with white ermine and satin.

"You always mount so gracefully?" drawled the barbarian.

She shot him a shriveling glare and looked away disdainfully. "I am accustomed to the aid of a groom."

Then her eyes cut back at him askance. It now occurred to the Imperial Princess that for the first time in her life she was alone with a man—no maids, nurses, or guards—and, moreover, alone not with a nobleman of gentle birth, but a savage warrior of perhaps the most uncivilized race on Earth.

His bronze shoulders, glistening with sweat and sunlight, were a powerfully contoured mountain, slashed in half a dozen places with scarred ravines, the wounds of uncounted battles. His arms rippled with strength beneath garnet-and-gold armbands and wristbands. A torque of twisted gold and silver encircled the muscle-corded neck, and yellow hair hung wild and tangled about his chiseled profile. His features were rugged and severe, the dark blue eyes predatory and hawk-like beneath the craggy brows.

Dia's heart raced in sudden unaccountable panic, and she felt her pulse throbbing in the hollow of her throat. She swallowed quickly and bent her attention studiously to her mare, patting the sweaty white neck.

He rode too close, she thought, and though she was not quite sure why that disturbed her, she reined the mare toward the highway. With relief she saw that they would soon be meeting the vanguard of the Gothic cavalcade.

If Dia had been able to read Atawulf's mind, she would have been even more alarmed, for his glance slid lingeringly in her direction. The image of her lithe form leaning into the jump as the mare leapt brush and driftwood, the thin blue shift billowing around her knees—that image would tantalize him for many a night.

"What are you staring at?"

"You told the truth about one thing. You *can* ride."

"You sound surprised."

"I am," he said with exaggerated astonishment. "Why, who would've thought you'd ride so well for a—"

"For a Roman?"

"I didn't say that."

"But you thought it."

True, Atawulf had been about to say that very thing, but she annoyed him, unreasonably so, and he was equally annoyed with himself for letting her get under his skin.

"In fact, I didn't expect you to ride so well for a spoiled, pampered, nose-in-the-air Roman princess."

"I am *not*—" Dia sucked in a furious breath and fought for dignity. "I am the daughter of Theodosius—"

"The resemblance is uncanny," he said dryly. " 'Tis the temper, I think."

"Thank you," she countered. "My father taught me to ride." She half smiled, and the soft expression made her look as sweet and appealing as the little girl her father had adored. "My earliest memory of Papa is going riding with him. He would sit me before him on his horse—I was very small, no more than three years old—he'd put his big arm around me, holding me safe, and off we'd trot. And for my fourth birthday he gave me my own pony. I remember how much I loved our riding lessons." Her voice wavered a little.

"I saw you with him. He introduced you to the legions."

"I remember. The Goths howled like a pack of wolves."

"Aye, that would be us. I happen to recall that when we set off to war, a little girl leaned off the terrace and howled. She wouldn't have been you, would she, Miss Protocol?"

Dia stared at him, surprised. "And the grinning warrior with the black wolf's head . . . ?"

"Bold Wolf," he grinned.

"Oh, my. I was only five."

"Aye, a woman dragged you back."

Oh, she had not forgotten. Serena.

"I don't remember," she said, her eyes slipping away from his, skimming past him to the paved road. "In any case, it was an inexcusable breach of pro——"

"Woman, I don't want to hear another word about protocol."

Dia laughed lightly. "Oh, you should've been raised at court."

"No," said Atawulf seriously. "I shouldn't. I grew up with my people. My da sat me on my first horse, put the first shield into my hands, showed me how to swing my first wooden sword. He taught me what it is to be a warrior. Da was one of the best, and the only regret I remember as a boy is that he was off to war so much . . ."

Dia nodded, knowing that feeling well.

Bold Wolf's words trailed off. Dia's gaze was clear and glistening. Her eyes, fringed with dark lashes, were as cool and deep and inviting as a spring-fresh forest pool.

He forgot the trail of his thoughts and she never noticed. She noticed only that his eyes were like summer thunderclouds lit by the sunlight of his face, and little crinkles at the corners of his eyelids looked like laughter. They were the eyes of the boy become the man, with all the spirit of freedom and hardship and hope and life in them—of loss and of love.

Their mounts had come to a standstill, and so, it seemed, had the rest of the world around them—stilled and silenced while their gazes touched, their eyes clear and unveiled in the shimmering sunlight.

Suddenly, with a visible start, Dia pulled her gaze away, darted her glance to the weedy ground, to the rocks, to anything but the face of the man beside her. Feeling the hot flush on her cheeks, she turned her face away, furious with herself. What traitorous turn was this, that her soul could be drawn in by those barbarian eyes?

She dared not look at Atawulf, who she was sure would be wearing a mocking grin.

In truth, Atawulf was staring at her with bemused fascination—as much bemused by his own reaction as hers. What had prompted the sudden vulnerability, this inviting discovery with which she regarded him, and what was he to do with it? It was one thing to tease this beautiful, haughty woman—quite another to fall under her spell. If it *was* vulnerability and not some play on his sympathy; she possessed a dangerous arsenal of feminine charms, and it disturbed the Bold Wolf to discover he was not immune to them. He should never let himself forget she was a Roman—worse, an Imperial.

With an uneasy sense of relief he heard his name shouted as the cavalcade caught up with them, and the two of them rode back to the highway in potent silence.

5

For the hundredth time Dia pummeled the silken pillow as though it alone kept her awake. She flung herself from stomach to side, then to her back. The coverlet had hours ago been kicked to the coach floor; the thin nightshift twisted about her restless legs.

Tiny irritating rivulets of sweat trickled down her limbs, and the sultry air lay heavy as a blanket upon her body.

She sighed her frustration into the black oven, blaming her sleeplessness on the heat, knowing with growing anger that was but half the truth.

He's a savage. A barbarian. How could I ever have forgotten that, even for an instant?

It's that grin of his, that brash, self-assured grin and those laughing eyes.

He is the enemy of all I hold sacred. The enemy of all civilization. He's a warrior. It's his trade.

He's a marauder. He attacks and kills unarmed citizens of the Empire.

He saved me from the ravages of that beast.

Only because I'm the Imperial Princess. But for that he might have raped me himself.

He doesn't seem like the others.

He's one of them, this pack of savages. Only a traitor's heart would find excuses for him.

I am no traitor. He is my enemy, and the enemy of everything good and decent. I despise everything he is.

Never be such a fool as to forget that again.

Never.

Near dawn she fell asleep, only to be awakened by the early stirrings of the Gothic camp. She quarreled with Dulcie and snapped at Thalia, and Dulcie, bold as a barbarian, dared talk about her before her very face.

"Oh, she's in a mood this morning," clucked Dulcie, nodding at Thalia. " 'Twill be that Atawulf, I'll bet, who put her into it."

"Dulcie, my moods are no business of yours."

"Aye, a handsome one he is, too, with those smoldering eyes. And the way he looks at a woman!" Dulcie roved her gaze in imitation of Atawulf, glancing slyly at Dia. "Hard for a young woman who hasn't been kissed in two years, you know, to resist eyes like that."

Dia drew herself up primly. "I am having no trouble resisting his eyes, I'll have you know. And you'll hold your tongue, girl."

"You see," Dulcie nodded, ignoring the warning, "just talking about him makes her angry. A sure sign, if you ask me—"

Thalia shook her head warningly. "Dulcie—"

"—that she's taken to him and won't admit it."

Dia was on her feet now. "You're asking for a lashing, girl!"

"And who's going to try it?" Dulcie shot back at her.

Dia gasped. Her hand shot out, and she struck blindly in her frustration and misery at the gadfly that was her maid.

But Dulcie was quicker; the woman caught Dia's arm, halting the slap in midair.

"You've no right hitting me, Miss Dia," Dulcie reproved her. "I've done nothing but speak my mind, that's all."

Dia jerked her wrist from the larger woman's grasp. "How dare you lay a hand on me! Slaves have died for less."

Dulcie rose to her feet, smoothing her limp dress with surprising dignity, her fair complexion reddened with anger. "I've been laying hands on you all your life, you're forgetting. Patting and oiling and powdering, doing your hair up fancy, painting your toes, draping your fine garments, and I never heard no objections neither. And I don't have to be here neither! I figured you'd be glad to have me, Miss Noble Princess. But you have to treat me with respect for what I am now—a free woman of the Goths."

Dia's eyes narrowed. "A traitor to Rome, you mean."

Dulcie's blue eyes flared. "To Rome I'm nothing but state property, same as my mother was. She gave the state seven babies before she died—seven slave babies—and not a one of them she could call her own. Me, I've been careful not to have babies. I'm not as wanton as you believe, missy, and I've watched my moontime and used vinegar sponges and rose-hip purges, but now—now I don't need to, you see, because now my babies will be born free. They may be what you call barbarians, but they'll be free among their own kind!"

She clutched up her skirts and jerked open the coach door. "So don't call me a traitor, Miss Imperial Princess, because I don't owe Rome no loyalty, nor do I owe you, and if you can't be civil to me, why, you can bloody well do without me."

Wounded dignity on her round pink face, Dulcie descended the fold-down steps and slammed the coach door behind her.

Dia stared after her in astonishment, and then with mounting fury. She rounded on Thalia, whose eyes were black orbs of astonishment themselves.

"What are *you* staring at, girl?"

The Greek slave dropped her gaze hastily, but not hastily

enough for her mistress. All the fury and misery and frustration raging through Dia found their victim. The slap Dia had meant for Dulcie struck Thalia full across the face.

Thalia turned away, hand pressed to her cheek, not daring to move or glance up. Dia stood before her, shaking. In all her life, Dia had never struck Thalia; it hardly seemed possible that she had done it now.

Dia swallowed convulsively. What was done . . . was done.

"That was for listening!" she snapped at her maid. "And in case you're thinking of being so bold as to speak above your station—well, you'll remember your place from now on."

Thalia did not look up. Her voice sounded dull and far away. "Yes, nobilissima."

Dia clenched both fists. Why did she not feel vindicated in her self-righteous tantrum? Why did she feel so spiteful? So defeated? So helplessly trapped in circumstances out of her control?

She could not bear the confines of the coach another second, nor the unspoken reproach in Thalia's downcast eyes and rigid shoulders. She shoved angrily at the door and fumbled her way down the steps into the soft glow of a misty dawn, refreshingly cool after the stuffy interior of the coach. She inhaled a delightful breath of clean air fragrant with the sea. It reminded her of lovely trips to the seashore with her aunts, and made her feel homesick.

One of the omnipresent guards met her before both sandals touched ground, and, as usual, she paid him no attention. Tired from her restless night, she sat on the lower step and shivered slightly, surprised that she needed a light cloak this morning. But she could not bring herself to call to Thalia for a wrap, picturing the black hair shadowing her maid's lowered face, her narrow shoulders hunched and stiffened. She would not ruin her morning with Thalia's sulks. Besides, Dia told herself uncomfortably, Thalia might mistake an invitation outside for a relenting on her mistress's part, and Dia had no intention of relenting. It never hurt to remind a slave of her place.

"Up on the wrong side of the bed, Your Royalty?"

Her head snapped up. Atawulf stood grinning down at her, with that lazy, teasing grin. A decidedly irritating grin, she thought.

"I beg your pardon?"

"Did you have a bad night, or do you always get up this cheerful?"

"My night is no business of yours, nor am I obliged to be cheerful in the mornings."

Atawulf stepped back and raised his hands as though under attack. "Pardon me, Your Graciousness, for being so thoughtless as to inquire after your welfare."

"I doubt that my welfare is of serious interest to you."

"Oh, how I enjoy having my head bitten off first thing in the morning. That's the real reason I came calling, not to extend an invitation from a most gracious Gothic noblewoman to breakfast with her."

"Oh . . . well . . . to breakfast? I suppose I must accept, mustn't I?"

"No," growled Atawulf, "but she won't ask twice."

"You needn't take offense so easily," Dia told him hastily. The truth be known, no one had extended her any kind of invitation at all, and the Imperial Princess had begun to feel slighted, even if they were only Goths.

"I meant I *should* accept her invitation in the interest of diplomacy. Is she a very important noblewoman?"

Atawulf grinned again. "The *most* important. You should feel deeply honored, Princess."

Dia reddened, not knowing whether to be angry because he was mocking her or because he insinuated that meeting some barbarian woman could possibly be considered an honor to Roman royalty.

Stiffly Dia rose to her feet, ignoring Atawulf's offered hand. "Very well. Shall I expect some sort of conveyance?"

"No, we'll walk. It isn't far."

"What—now?"

"Of course, now. You wouldn't be so inconsiderate as to keep her waiting."

Before Dia could reply his broad hand closed about her arm and propelled her along beside him. Indignantly she attempted to shake him off.

"Let go of me. I'm perfectly capable of walking by myself. Or are you afraid I'm going to run away again?"

Atawulf released his grip abruptly.

"Try it," he drawled amiably.

She rubbed her arm and allowed him a wry smile. "Without my breakfast? No, thank you. But after breakfast—watch out."

He laughed then, a rowdy shout of pure enjoyment, and might have flung an arm about her shoulders if he had not known full well he would be angrily rebuffed. As it was, he turned a face wreathed in amusement to hers, then, with a tilt of his head, invited her to walk alongside him.

Damn those wicked blue eyes, Dia warned her fluttering heart. *He's doing it again.*

As the two of them passed tents and wagons whose sleepy occupants were coaxing morning fires to life, Dia realized that something was different about the routine of the Gothic caravan. No one was hitching mules and oxen to the scattered wagons; no one folded tents or bundled belongings. Indeed, the camp seemed half deserted.

"Aren't we moving on today?" wondered Dia.

"No."

"No? Why not?"

"We took Anxur last night; today we load up our plunder."

"You sacked the town." Dia's voice shook with disgust. Anxur must have been the seacoast town she glimpsed down the beach yesterday, the town in which she briefly hoped she might reach sanctuary. No chance of that now.

"I knew you'd object."

"Object! I abhor it—detest it! I detest you! You and your pretenses at being so civilized, *so* solicitous of my welfare, *so* pleasant—the benevolent conqueror—"

"At least you admit we're the conquerors."

"All the time you're nothing but a savage—a beast in man's clothing!"

"Even a beast must attack to survive. We have thousands to feed."

"I shudder to think of those poor people, set upon in the night, defenseless against the swords of your bloodthirsty—"

"Half of those people fled before we were within fifty miles. Those who stayed surrendered readily enough."

"And you doubtless robbed them of everything they owned, leaving them nothing."

"Their lives. We left them their lives."

"And with no food left in the storehouses, they'll starve."

Atawulf shrugged. "Better them than us."

"Oh! You are despicable!"

Atawulf spun her about, his flint-blue eyes hard and glinting. "Do you think the Roman Legions never sacked a town, Miss Too-Holy-to-Piss? The Empire is built on sacked towns and trampled nations and slaughtered children. And you—you Imperials on Palatine Hill live in luxury on the plunder and labor of conquered peoples who fought Rome every blood-slick step of the way."

Dia glared back at him in fury. "You dare compare the conquests of the Roman Empire to your rampant banditry—your wanton destruction! Rome had purpose and vision, if those people could but see it! Rome was *building* a civilization; the Goths are *destroying it!*"

"No one ever wanted your civilization!"

Dia's lips curved into a sharp little scythe of a smile. "Oh, really? Then I must be mistaken in my notion that you Goths arrived—uninvited, I recall—on our borders and *begged to be allowed into the Empire!*"

"My, my," interjected a husky feminine voice. "I can see we're in for a pleasant breakfast this morning."

Two gazes that could have sheared iron turned on the source of the richly amused voice. She was a tall, elderly woman; iron-grey hair brushed her hips in thick braids intertwined with dyed, glass-beaded leather. She was old as an oak tree is old, her face sun-bronzed and wrinkled, the pale blue eyes crystal-clear and lively.

She wore a skirt layered with festival hues of colored wool. A triple-stranded necklace of gold inlaid with carnelian, turquoise, and jet lay upon the breast of a simple bright blue overtunic. Bracelets of enameled design decorated her bare freckled arms.

"Mother."

Dia's startled gaze swung to Atawulf and then back to the barbarian woman.

"Your mother?"

"The gracious lady herself."

Dia brushed back a wayward strand of hair. It was certainly not proper etiquette to be caught arguing with the son of the woman she was about to have breakfast with.

"You might have warned me!" she hissed at him before she stepped regally forward.

The grey-haired woman smiled. "Warned you of what? That I'm a formidable old crow? Don't believe it. I'm glad you came, Princess Placidia."

The woman's smile was friendly, but Placidia noticed that, like everyone else in the Gothic camp, she made no move to show the proper respect due the Imperial Princess.

Absolutely no one ever bows, Dia sighed to herself, but she met the smile with a polite one of her own.

"No, he might have warned me that the noblewoman who invited me to breakfast was his mother. And the foster mother of Ala—— King Alaric, I believe."

The lady inclined her head. "I am Singledia."

Before Dia finished murmuring her polite, "I'm pleased to

make your—" the woman was already striding away, her steps long and sure in boots of toughened red leather.

"Come along."

Dia had to hurry to catch up to the older woman, stumbling on the rocky ground in her woven silk sandals of gold and purple. Atawulf fell into step beside Dia, favoring her with a lopsided grin—at her expense, she suspected.

They followed Singledia to one of the largest tents Dia had seen in the camp. It was made of the dyed oxhide favored by the Goths, and colorful figures of wolves and hawks decorated the outside. From the simple triangular tent in the center, wings stretched to either side, forming an interior spacious enough to live in comfortably. Most of that interior was on view, both front flaps of the large central area pulled fully open, so that the tent was flooded with the warmth and light of the morning sun.

Dia followed the woman inside, curious. The only pieces of furniture were a simple folding camp chair of carved cedarwood and a trunk of the same, but the whole of the floor was carpeted with furs so numerous they were laid overlapping, so varied they were strewn like a scattered mosaic of rabbit and fox, beaver and otter, muskrat, bear, and wolf.

Bundles of belongings hung from pegs on the interior poles, and a deep pile of furs under one of the wings made a bed soft, warm, and dry.

Singledia bade them be seated beside an expensive purple-and-silver linen cloth—taken from the Great Palace in Rome, Dia realized with sudden recognition—and they sat upon the fur-strewn floor. Atawulf, and Singledia in her full skirts, sank at once to cross-legged positions, but Dia tucked her feet modestly to the side, the simple contours of her silk-pleated skirt not allowing her the barbarian woman's freedom. Besides, she had been taught that ladies did not sit cross-legged in any circumstance.

"I wished to invite you, Placidia," the barbarian woman said, "when we could sit down to a proper meal, but who knows when that will be. I expect you're accustomed to a fancier breakfast than cold cheese and grapes on the run. These youngsters"—she waved at Atawulf—"are in such a hurry, it's 'Put up the tent, take down the tent; pack, unpack; hitch the mules, unhitch the mules.' Won't say where we're off to, either."

Dia shook her head and tore into warmed-over hard bread, dipping a chunk into olive oil simmering in a silver bowl. "I adore cold cheese and grapes for breakfast—especially in summer—and bread and oil. Thank you for inviting me, Lady . . . Singledia. I'm grateful for the change of scenery; I'm rather tired of traveling in that stuffy old coach."

"So I've heard." Singledia grinned, missing only a couple of teeth. "I understand you went riding yesterday. Has my Atawulf been treating you right?"

Dia's dark lashes raised, and she gazed at the woman in startled surprise. Hastily she swallowed her mouthful.

"Why, yes, I . . . he was . . . *is* very considerate . . . considering." She glanced at Atawulf, then looked quickly away.

"Mother," grumbled Atawulf, "I know how to treat a wo— um, a woman of . . . royal sensibilities."

"Just what is that supposed to mean?" Dia inquired, those royal sensibilities detecting a note of condescension.

"Nothing. You're just accustomed to more pampering and fussing over than your average woman."

"Well, I'll have you know that does not make me one whit less able to stand up to a difficult journey. I daresay I could endure the same treatment as any other woman in this caravan!"

"Oh?" Atawulf's intense gaze held challenge, and a half-teasing suggestion that he might enjoy testing her assertion to the fullest.

Blushing, Dia suddenly pretended great interest in her breakfast.

His mother, Atawulf realized, listened to this exchange with sharp glances between Dia and himself. Suddenly he, too, demonstrated great fascination in breakfast.

The old woman pursed her weathered lips together in thought. So her son had not taken her riding yesterday simply for the exercise.

"Well," Singledia said sagely, "these boys of mine, oh, they're great movers of armies—horses and men—but when it comes to the care and comfort of a delicate little thing like yourself—"

Dia set her winecup down abruptly.

"I *do* wish people would stop referring to me as a delicate little thing or a . . . a quivering mass of royal sensibilities!"

Atawulf choked behind his cup.

"In fact, Lady Singledia, I am being positively smothered with comforts and considerations. Living inside that 'luxury' coach is a torment."

Dia stopped suddenly, realizing even her protestations sounded like a spoiled little girl's complaints. She smiled, and the mischievous little girl danced in her sea-green eyes.

"Though, if you could arrange it, broiled turbot in cream sauce would be nice."

Atawulf snorted, spewing wine across the tablecloth.

"Atawulf!" his mother rapped sharply.

Helplessly the Bold Wolf shook his head. "Hoo! Ma, I'm sorry. I'll be good, I swear."

"Humph." Singledia indicated her disbelief. She turned with penetrating scrutiny to the princess.

"So, we're providing you with too many comforts. First time I ever heard a complaint like that."

"I . . . it's not exactly *too many* amenities . . . it's just not exactly the right ones."

The old woman's crystalline blue eyes studied her critically, causing Dia to feel flustered, as though she was found wanting.

"The trouble with you, girl, is you're spoiled. Everything always perfect. All the amenities, is it? Always gotten your way, haven't you?"

Stunned at this unwarranted attack, Dia could only stare at the woman in disbelief. Then, unexpectedly, tears sprang into her eyes. Tired, sleepless, unwashed, upset for having slapped Thalia in a temper, and now attacked by this wretched old barbarian crone—it was all too much.

"No, I haven't always had my way! You don't know—you've no right to judge me and my life! You don't know anything about me!"

Dia fought back angry tears, tears over all those tragedies which she would give anything to change—Mama dying; and Papa; and Serena, haughty, hateful Serena making her childhood miserable; Elpidia left behind in Rome—oh, how she missed her dear nurse and friend; and now this . . . this wretched journey, captive to barbarians, wondering what they were finally going to do with her . . .

"You don't know how much I've *never* had my way!" She bit the words off angrily, fighting the trembling in her voice. "Just because I've been accustomed to a few luxuries you think my life's been too perfect, don't you? Now it's time to bring the haughty princess down from her high and mighty palace! Well, you're too late, you Goths—this is just one more thing I never wanted to happen, just one more journey from one misery to another, just one more senseless cruelty God has flung in my face—and I wish I knew . . . I wish I knew what I did to make him hate me so!"

She hiccupped loudly and wiped at her teary eyes with the back of her hand, embarrassed and miserable. She did not see the look-what-you've-done glare Atawulf threw at his mother. Singledia blithely ignored his frown, gazing with renewed interest and apparent delight at the young woman struggling to sniffle back her tears.

"We're not out to make your life miserable, Galla Placidia, no matter what you think," the barbarian woman told her. "Don't you know why you're here?"

"Because I was unlucky enough to be in your path."

"Well, aye, that's true enough. But we brought you with us because we need a bargaining point with the Emperor."

"I know," Dia said wearily. "I'm just a pawn—*again*," she added bitterly, thinking of Serena.

"You know, girl, you're too old to be a weepy child. Be a woman. Be a warrior!"

"What?" Dia's voice cracked, hysteria tightening her throat.

"We women have to be strong. We face as much hardship as men in our time, and we face it like warriors in our own way. Be strong, be fearless—be a warrior."

"A warrior," Dia repeated slowly, deliberately, staring at the tough old woman as though she were mad. "You want me to take up a sword and do battle?"

"*I've* done it, make no mistake," Singledia told her sternly. "But you don't have to wield a sword to be a warrior. It takes courage and strength and pride to be a warrior, and if you haven't those—courage, strength, and pride—then by what right are you a princess of the Romans?"

Startled, Dia raised her eyes to the gaze regarding her from a lifetime of hardship. The barbarian woman might have been Elpidia speaking. At least she was saying those very things Elpidia would be reminding her of, if her old nurse were here. Elpidia would not let her forget she was the daughter of emperors, would not let her sink into self-pity.

She sniffed one last time, lifted her chin, and drew back her small shoulders, managing to look stubborn and vulnerable and regal all at once.

Atawulf, despite earlier warnings to himself, felt his heart leap toward this royal woman-child; for she had been so sheltered and pampered all her life, she seemed a child in many ways, but there was no mistaking the woman. That sensuous lift of her head, the easy, flowing grace with which she moved, the way her eyes sometimes met his with stirring vitality—he saw that woman now, beautiful, determined, proud.

"I apologize for my outburst, Lady Singledia. I . . . it's been a . . . a tiring journey . . . I had quite a shock, being abducted from my bed by an army . . . You're right, of course . . . the daughter of Theodosius should meet adversity without self-pity or tears . . ."

"You did fine," growled Atawulf, "until my mother got her talons into you."

". . . these little setbacks, like being held hostage by a hostile army . . ."

"Bold Wolf," Singledia snapped, "that is no way to talk to your old mother."

". . . an army of sworn enemies to my people . . . to my brother . . ."

"I have to do my poking and prodding," Singledia went on, ignoring the murmuring princess. "You know my way of testing a person's edge."

". . . a barbarian king who's sworn to destroy my whole civilization . . ."

"Setting their nerves on edge, you mean," said Atawulf. "You're a meddler. What's your sudden interest anyway? Why did you really invite Dia here?"

"*Dia,* is it now?"

". . . really, why should I be in the least upset . . . how silly of me . . ."

"Mother, you're meddling."

". . . acting like a spoiled child . . . I've only been dragged from my burning city and carried away by a band of barbarians . . ."

"Are you forgetting, Atawulf—she's a *Roman!* Sister to the Emperor!"

". . . daughter of Theodosius, don't forget . . . granddaughter of . . ."

"*Dia!*" Atawulf grasped her by the shoulders and turned her toward him, fearing perhaps his mother had actually, at last, driven someone mad. "Stop it! Dia!"

Furiously she shoved at his hands and twisted away from his grasp. "I forbid you to call me that. Marauder! Abductor!" She turned her glare next upon Singledia. "Do not presume to tell me how to behave. It is your sons who have kidnapped me, your people who hold me hostage. I have done nothing to warrant your criticism—and I certainly do not require you to tell me how a royal princess should behave!"

Singledia, to Dia's astonishment, clapped her hands together and rocked backward with laughter. Low, throaty chortles met Dia's ire and knocked it flat. She could only stare, perplexed.

"Imperial to the bone!" crowed the old woman, in that raspy, strangely musical voice. She crooked a work-roughened finger at the startled princess. "Told me off right and proper, you did. That's good, that's good. Be a warrior. Fight back."

Dia's gaze shifted from mother to son, but Atawulf met her eyes with a shrug of his massive shoulders and a droll raising of his brows in a what-can-I-do-she's-my-mother expression.

Singledia reached out and tugged sharply at his long fair hair. "Ow!"

"Don't make faces behind your old ma's back, son."

"I wasn't behind your back, you wicked crow. Why make faces if you can't see 'em?"

Dia could not help smiling to herself; the sight of this iron-muscled warrior of the Goths bantering with his spirited, shrewd-tongued old mother was too incongruous. At the same time she felt a pang of loneliness, a yearning for Elpidia, who was as close as she had to a mother, and whose sturdy love she missed terribly. So her smile was a small one and a little sad.

Singledia's sharp eyes missed nothing.

"You going to cry again?"

Hastily Dia shook her head.

"Feeling a bit homesick, I expect."

"A bit."

"I can't send you home, you know that, but if there's anything I can do to make it a little easier . . ."

Dia shook her head, but then something occurred to her. She leaned forward and spoke in a confidential tone to the old woman, who reminded her so much of Elpidia, of whom she could have asked anything.

"Well, there is *one* thing—"

"Da! Da!" Happy voices shrilled into the tent as a whole pack of young barbarians raced in.

"Da!"

"Uncle Wolf!"

The youngest two, a boy and a girl, flung themselves upon Atawulf, who yelped and toppled backward, then rolled about the floor howling with laughter as the youngsters worried at him like a couple of pups.

The two older girls, however, were quick to turn their attention to the visitor.

"Who's this, Gran?"

"Is she the Roman? The princess?"

"Is she?"

"Aye, she is," said Singledia. "If you'll be quiet long enough, I'll introduce you."

Dia saw that the two girls were young ladies in their teens, perhaps twelve and fourteen. Their attire was colorful and bangled, much like their grandmother's, and they wore their fair hair in long, thick braids. Bold eyes and curious expressions faced Dia expectantly.

"Galla Placidia," beamed Singledia, "my granddaughters—Singledia and Alfreya."

Dia inclined her head regally, and the girls nodded back, imitating her poised reserve. They were certainly no more impressed with her royalty than anyone else, but Dia quickly realized why.

"They're Alaric's and Winnifreya's daughters," Singledia told her, raising her raspy voice above the din created by Atawulf wrestling with his two shrieking attackers.

That would be *King* Alaric and *Queen* Winnifreya to the Goths, Dia remembered. These girls were royal princesses of this barbarian tribe, which was no status at all to an Imperial Princess of Rome, but she knew enough of diplomatic protocol not to hint at the disparity in their ranks.

"Princesses," Dia acknowledged gravely, just as the trio of wrestlers rolled onto the linen cloth, knocking bowls and goblets asunder. A girl's squeals and a boy's delighted shouts of triumph, aided by Atawulf's bellowing laughter, made a shambles of the remains of breakfast, and it was some moments before the tickling, thumping battle was called a truce. Atawulf emerged with a beard streaked with wine; he held a feisty little boy at arm's length, who had to be persuaded to give up the fight.

Growling good-naturedly, Atawulf called the tow-headed children to order and introduced them to Dia.

"Athelwulf, my son," he said, and a boy of about six years looked up at her with a bright grin that matched his father's in charm and mischief.

"Hello, Athelwulf," she managed to answer. She had not known he had children, and for some reason the knowledge disconcerted her. What could it possibly matter to her that this Goth had children?

"Amalasuntha, my daughter."

These barbaric names, she despaired, but she stumbled over the girl's name as best she could. The girl, who was about eight or nine years old, giggled at her shyly.

"Go on, now, children, all of you." Singledia waved her hands as though to shoo them out. "I want to talk to Placidia, and I can't hear myself with a gaggle of grandchildren running about. You, too, Bold Wolf—you've done enough damage to breakfast for one morning. Go along."

"Come on, Da!" The boy tugged at his father's hand. "You'll stay and play with us, won't you?"

"Please!" The little girl forgot Dia in an instant.

"I'll tell you what," said Atawulf, "let's see how you two are at riding nowdays."

"I can ride!"

"Me, too!"

"Well, 'tis time I saw how good you are, isn't it? Why, my da had me up on a war-horse when I was your age, Athel."

"Can I ride a war-horse, too?" the girl wanted to know as they herded their father out of the tent.

"No, but I have a pretty white mare I save especially for beautiful princesses." Atawulf winked at Dia over his daughter's head and turned away, a child swinging on each hand.

Singledia shooed the older girls out behind them and then surveyed the damage to her tent. Dia stared out into the sunlight, watching Atawulf and his two children until they turned out of her sight. She had never imagined him as a father; it seemed strange to discover that he had two children who adored him, children he wrestled and laughed with. Children were a bit of a mystery to Dia; she had rarely been in their company.

"Where is their mother?" Dia asked the woman.

"Dead."

"Oh. I'm sorry."

Singledia regarded her measuredly. "You have your sights set on my son?"

"Why, hardly!" Dia was surprised. "I scarcely know him. And beyond the fact that he's a . . . an enemy of my people and that he abducted me . . . beyond that, I don't want to know."

"Good. Best kept that way, I say, between Goths and Romans."

"At least we are in agreement about something."

"Aye."

The two women stood in silence, the older soberly assessing the younger, the younger imperiously defying her to find fault.

"Imperial as hell," Singledia judged, nodding.

"I beg your—"

"But not fit to rule . . . yet. Oh, you've got the fire for it, but not the wisdom, not the heart."

"Why, I don't know who you think you—"

"It may come—or maybe not. Depends on what you're made of, Galla Placidia."

For once Dia was speechless. She fidgeted with her skirt, then she shrugged. "Well, I won't have to worry about that. An Imperial Princess does not become Empress unless she marries an Emperor—and both emperors are my half-brothers, so there is no question of me ruling—that's impossible."

"But you'd jump at it, given the chance, wouldn't you?"

"Yes, of course . . . I . . . no!" Her jade-blue eyes hardened with suspicion. "Are you trying to trick me into some kind of treason? As Alaric did Priscus Attalus? You'll not use me as a puppet to depose my brother!"

Singledia shook her head. "Aye, you're that quick to anger, you are. I'm just talk, you know. Full of an old woman's notions. Now, there was something you wanted to ask of me earlier—before the grandchildren ran in—what was it, girl?"

"I . . . well, I can't ask Atawulf, because he thinks it's silly and needless, but . . . Lady Singledia, I'd give anything for a chance to bathe—oh, and wash my hair, and have my clothes clean. You see, I've started my blood-flow—"

"I *thought* you were touchy."

"—and now that we've come to the sea . . ." Dia looked at Singledia questioningly. "Don't Gothic women ever feel the need to bathe?"

"You think we don't wash? You Romans think we live in filth and horse dung, don't you?"

"Well, not precisely . . ."

"We wash! It just happens there's scarcely enough water in this parched country to wet your tongue—and all extra water goes for the horses and cattle. You'll see folk down at the seashore today, washing for all they're worth."

"I'd be grateful if I could join them."

Singledia nodded. "I'll see to it. If you want to get ready, I'll have guards take you back to your coach."

Dia took her leave of the woman with a lighter heart than she had felt in her entire captivity. Followed closely by the guards she returned to the coach and informed Thalia they were going down to the sea to bathe.

"And gather the clothes that need washing," she ordered the maid.

Wordlessly Thalia began stuffing garments into a basket, not looking at her mistress. Dia had not forgotten about slapping her. She really should never have lost her temper that way, Dia knew; she was brought up to value gravity and dignity, and that did not include losing self-control in tantrums. Violent emotional scenes were unbecoming and uncivilized, as all the old philosophers taught. Besides, she felt ashamed at having struck out at Thalia, who was innocent, really, of anything beyond being in her way when she was angry.

Dia sighed. One simply could not apologize to a slave. It was not done. It was rather silly of her to feel the need to make amends at all.

But Thalia had been at her side as long as she could remember, through everything, growing up with her, listening to her troubles and joys, sharing the cheerful times and the fearful times. This wall of silence in place of their easy companionship hurt more than Dia cared to admit.

She watched Thalia finish filling the basket and turn to pack stringents and oils for bathing. As though she could feel her mistress's gaze on her, Thalia glanced up; her dark eyes were moist with recently shed tears, but her face was carefully composed, devoid of animation or emotion.

That tore at Dia's heart more than anything, that stranger's expression on Thalia's familiar features. The slave bent back to her task, straight black hair veiling her face.

"Thalia, I . . . I shall wear an undergarment for bathing, and so must you. We'll have no privacy from the men."

There, she had invited her maid to bathe; she had come as close to an apology as she dared. Thalia would understand that, surely.

"Yes, mistress," Thalia said tonelessly.

"You . . . you might at least be pleased that we're finally going to get a bath after this sweltering journey."

"I am pleased, mistress," her maid dutifully agreed.

"Well, you don't *act* pleased!"

Thalia looked up, and this time there were flashes of emotion in those inky pools—anger, perhaps, and pain.

"I will *act* however you wish me to act, miss, if I know what that is. I hope you will forgive me if I am not accustomed to *acting*."

"There! You're angry with me. I know you are. You're being sarcastic. You're always sarcastic when you're angry."

Thalia looked quickly away, blinking her eyes. "It is not for me to be angry with you, nobilissima."

Dia felt like an ogre, and she did not like the feeling. Too many things were happening that were out of her control, and if she had to endure another moment of this thoroughly distant Thalia she was going to be near tears.

"You're doing this to me on purpose, Thalia. It's to make me feel bad for slapping you this morning. Well, all right, I feel bad." To her dismay, those tears threatened. "I forbid you to make me feel any worse."

Thalia peered at her obliquely from behind a curtain of black hair. They had only each other, the Greek slave and the Roman princess. They were all the two of them had left of home, of the familiar, of that lost life that had seemed so safe and secure, of childhood.

The Greek maid's face melted into a quirky little smile, and she swept straight strands of hair behind her ear with her habitual gesture.

"Mistress," she said with a hint of laughter, "you are a trial to your poor handmaiden, that's a fact."

Dia's relief was so great she felt a trembling in her lower lip. Silly to be so emotional, she chided herself, and especially over her maid. What had she feared? That Thalia would never speak to her again—at least not in the old companionable way? Nonsense.

Thalia would never be so mean. Dear Thalia never bore a grudge. Dia swallowed back the threatening tears and stilled the trembling of her lips with an extremely put-upon pout.

"Well, you are a trial to your poor princess, the truth be known. And you shouldn't be, not when everything's so terribly unbearable. I don't know if I can endure another moment of captivity, or the heat, or these Goths. Thalia, I had the most wretched breakfast this morning and an absolute grilling by the wickedest old woman . . ."

Thalia did not coax Dia out of her misery; that was not Thalia's way. She leaned one elbow on the basket of clothes and listened. She let Dia ramble on, her lively dark eyes wide with attention as she lent patient ears.

". . . and then he went off and left me with that old woman, who really despises me, I do believe, and it's no wonder I'm in just a terrible temper, is it?"

Thalia shook her head in sympathy, *real* sympathy despite her urge to shake the princess, for this was Dia, who took such little things to heart until she stumbled over the folly of it on her own.

Suddenly Dia laughed ruefully. "I *am* in a terrible temper, aren't I, Thalia?"

Thalia smiled. "Yes, miss, you are."

"I shall strive to improve it—you know, dignity and serenity and all. Why, that Singledia practically challenged my right to call myself princess, if you can imagine. Such audacity! But *she* doesn't care a fig over what I've been through—Oh, my God, I sound just like Serena, don't I?"

Thalia nodded gravely.

Dia grimaced. "Perhaps I should start again." Her fingers folded and unfolded the pleats in her skirt as she thought it over. "Singledia is a . . . a mother of warriors. She's old, but she doesn't really seem old. She told me I should be a warrior, not a weeping child. At first I thought it was barbarian nonsense, but she said that a woman who is a warrior has strength, courage, and pride (she didn't mean haughtiness, either), and if I don't possess those, why, I have no business calling myself a princess. As if the purple wasn't something I was born to."

Dia paused, her eyes focused on some far inner horizon, her fingers now still and linked across her knee. When she spoke, her voice was thoughtful, questing.

"I think there must be more to it than just those three things—strength, courage, and pride. I'm not sure, but it seems something's missing. But Singledia . . . I believe she meant I hadn't *earned* the right to rule—they do that among the Goths, you know. I tried to tell her I wasn't going to rule anyway, so it didn't matter. Singledia doesn't exactly rule, but she *is* a warrior, I think. Perhaps she knows . . . you know . . . something."

"Now you sound like Mistress Dia," Thalia told her. "Remember how your aunt Justa used to tell us there was wisdom to be learned from everyone, if you just looked for it?"

"I'd almost forgotten that. And remember when Aunt Grata accused Justa of having 'not a fig's worth of wisdom,' because she created that terrible scandal at Grata's first wedding by riding on the hunt with the men."

Thalia's eyes danced. "Oh, and Lady Justa answered, 'You're one to talk of scandal, Grata. What about you and that live-in architect who's young enough to be your son?' "

"Oh, my, yes," giggled Dia. "Then Aunt Grata said, 'You know very well, Justa, he's redoing my villa.' "

" 'For four years?' " Thalia sputtered in imitation of Lady Justa's indignation.

"What a fight they almost got into, until they noticed how avidly we two girls were listening."

Thalia laughed—she had a sharp, gleeful laugh—remembering the aunties with fondness and delight.

Dia caught her laughter and let loose with merry peals of her own.

Therefore, when the captain of their guard paused to rap on

the coach door, he hesitated a moment, his attention caught by the harmonious music of feminine merriment within.

A smile tugged at his beard.

Therefore, when Thalia and Dia answered the rap on their door, they met a grinning man, his eyes and face alight with the joy of the morning.

The walk down to the shore brought them into a growing procession of women and children toward the sea. Most of the women carried bundles of clothing. Dia walked apart from the chattering groups of women; Thalia followed closely, the basket of washing upon her hip. The music of female voices halted here and there as Dia's escort of guards passed near. Lash-veiled eyes looked her over.

Dia wore a simple white linen shift for bathing, but over it she had elegantly draped a voluminous aquamarine palla shot through with threads of silver and gold. The rich embroidery around the edges was patterned with starfishes and seashells.

She held her head high under the drape of palla that covered her hair and framed her face with a glittering border of exquisite handiwork. She had no idea what these women were saying in their crude Gothic tongue, but she was certain she was the subject of every conversation as heads turned and hands gestured her way.

Why couldn't she be allowed to bathe in private? Without curious stares and comments? She had no place among these barbarian women and their savage children.

As she approached the invitingly lapping waves, Dia turned suddenly to the friendly face of the guardsman who had stood smiling before their coach this morning.

"I simply cannot bathe with all these guards standing about gawking. Dismiss them at once."

The guard captain's friendly expression fell to one of discomfort. "I can't do that, Your Royalty . . . uh, sorry, I mean nobilissima. Atawulf would skin me alive if I let something happen."

"Do you think I'm going to swim out to sea and escape? I'll

have you know, Captain, I am not a courtesan to bathe for the titillation of onlookers!"

"I think we should remedy that," cut in a harsh voice. "I know *I* would pay for the spectacle."

Dia gasped and spun toward the dreaded voice. On horseback sat Sigeric, steel-eyed and leering through his thick red beard. Her cold, hard, relentless attacker in the palace garden, whose hands had roved and grasped at her flesh, who would have raped her with no more thought for her pain and terror than if she were a rabbit caught in a snare to be slaughtered for dinner.

Mounted and armored, Sigeric had two dozen or more of his regiment behind him. He nudged his horse toward her, and Dia stumbled backward in panic. He pushed his mount closer. Heart pounding, Dia staggered into the sea, the waves tugging the hem of her shift around her ankles.

His grin was savage and hungry. "I'll take over guard duty now, soldier. You missed out on the plunder this morning; go and have your pick, you and your men."

"No!" Dia tried to cry, but what she meant for a scream emerged a breathless whisper.

Thalia, who had dropped the basket when the horse stepped between herself and her mistress, looked frantically to their guardsman. The captain glowered, his pleasant face a hard mask of anger.

"Atawulf gives us our orders, Sigeric."

"I'm only trying to do you boys a favor." His grin grew ugly, and his hard eyes, savoring Dia's horror even as they roved over the folds of her garments, seemed to be pawing her.

Dia clutched the palla tighter about her, as if the fine silk could armor her against his intent.

Sigeric, to her terror, dismounted. "I'll watch the precious princess take her bath, with pleasure."

"You will *not!*" A woman's knife-edged voice sliced the air. Sigeric jerked his head around to find the source of irritation.

Queen Winnifreya stepped forth, tall, straight, and sure, from a gathering group of women. Sea breeze and sunlight made a shimmering corona and veil of her abundant golden hair, unbound and free. She stood barefoot, her dress of blue woad ungirded and loose, her bare sun-brown arms and neck unadorned, her winter-sky eyes unwavering and clear.

Even in that terrible moment Dia was struck with how much the queen resembled her mother Singledia. How alike they were! The old crone in her youth must have been just like this golden woman.

"Alaric gave the order that the Imperial Princess should be *protected* from the likes of you. In fact, he may have meant you particularly, Sigeric."

Sigeric swiveled his head in an exaggerated sweeping search of the beach. His words were a soft sneer. "I don't see Atawulf anywhere. I feared he might have forgotten his duty and left a valuable hostage to the mercies of men less . . . *attentive*."

Dia heard an insinuation in the oily voice that seemed to give the word an ambiguous meaning, but the guardsmen, for their part, had no doubt of the slur upon both their war chief and themselves. Their stances tensed.

Winnifreya answered his charge. "Atawulf's duty is none of your concern, Sigeric. If you have none of your own, I suggest you ask Alaric where you might make yourself useful."

"Useful?" Sigeric almost spat, but thought better of it. "Where has Atawulf been while my men and I scoured the town for resistance, while we raided houses for plunder and set fire to the city, while we took captives for slaves? Or is Atawulf too squeamish for warrior's work?"

Sigeric's cold eyes raked over Dia once more, disdainfully. "Tell Atawulf we found plenty of women in town. I don't envy him a prize he can't enjoy. Or is Atawulf too squeamish for that kind of warrior's work, too?"

Winnifreya's eyes were glacial, but she did not answer immediately. Her first impulse was to tell the man he dared not say such things to Atawulf's face, but then, here in front of his men, he might take it as an accusation of cowardice. He would have no recourse but to insult Atawulf deliberately before witnesses. Then there would be fighting, which the Goths could ill afford to indulge in while on the move in the heart of Roman land. They must remain united.

The Queen of the Goths answered him levelly. "A warrior's work is *war*, Sigeric, in which my brother has no equal, excepting my husband. Atawulf fights with heart and courage, and none can stand against his sword. And while you enjoy the spoils, my brother sees to the war-horses and weapons, he looks to the warriors and their armor, and he trains the liberated Germanni to fight so that *you* might have a secure force behind you."

Now Sigeric did spit into the sand. "My horsemen don't *need* a lot of half-Roman curs at their backs."

"Perhaps Atawulf is thinking of the camp, the old and the wounded, women and children, who *do* need a sharp thicket of lances to defend them."

Confronted by a solid mass of solemn women, many of them holding babes in arms or clutching wide-eyed children tightly by the hand, Sigeric did not argue further.

He remounted his war-horse and, smiling, half mockingly touched his right fist to his breastplate in salute to his queen.

One last time his hard eyes lingered on Dia. Fear was a thing she could taste, fear and disgust, but she met his stare with a lift of her chin, with that royal aloofness that was so deeply ingrained in her that it stilled the trembling of her lips and hid the fear behind disdain.

Sigeric's parting words were for Dia's guardsmen. "Enjoy the view," he sneered. "That's all you'll get."

He jerked the reins of his mount around sharply and led his detachment down the beach at a canter.

Dia relaxed the fingers she clenched around the silky material of her palla and looked to Winnifreya. Humiliated, she stood in the ankle-deep tide and held her regal poise before her like a shield.

Queen Winnifreya took matters in hand. "Rayard," she told

the captain of the guard, "the princess will join me and my women. Your men may wait back from the shore with my own guard. The responsibility will be entirely mine if anything happens."

The guardsman inclined his head and saluted, clearly relieved that the queen was taking responsibility for the delicate situation he suddenly found himself in. He would hate to face Atawulf with the news that Sigeric or any other man, including himself, had looked on while Her Royalty bathed in the sea.

Dia lifted the wet hem of her shift and, trailing one corner of her palla in the water, slogged onto the beach with sandals heavy and slick and clogged with sand. She had to look up to meet the blue eyes of the tall Gothic woman.

"Thank you," she said only a little shakily. "I'm grateful."

"Not many of us would wish a similar encounter with Sigeric. Nor would we wish it on you, Princess."

Dia looked past Winnifreya to the women on the beach. Their stares were curious, but not unfriendly. A few even looked sympathetic, and those faces gave her a strange feeling of naked vulnerability, as though the women knew more of her fear and humiliation than she could bear. Quickly composing her features, she put on a dignified countenance.

She turned her attention from the other women to the queen. "Thank you, too, for the invitation. I accept."

Winnifreya smiled wryly. "It was a command, not an invitation. Besides, you weren't in a position to refuse."

"Yes. Queen Winnifreya, I think Atawulf should hear about this."

"Oh, he will hear of it, have no fear, probably before the morning is out."

"That man's conduct is reprehensible."

"Aye, it is, I agree." Winnifreya turned to include the women now beginning to surround them. "Most of us agree, do we not?"

The women chorused an accord.

"But," the queen said, "he is a valuable swordsman and has

a loyal following in his regiment. We need him, he and his ilk, whether we like his conduct or not."

"If Atawulf had been here," Dia said grimly, "he would not have gotten away with it."

"If Atawulf had been here," countered Winnifreya, "blood might have been shed. I'm glad he was not."

"Do you mean he will go unpunished?"

"Sigeric is a war chief. We cannot afford to split the chiefs and their men over one incident."

"Is not Alaric king? They have to obey him, do they not?"

"Aye, but he does not punish his warriors as though they were errant children. Alaric is king because the warriors believe in him, because he is the best among them and every man of them will follow him into battle. They do not follow him because he is king; he is king because they follow him."

The queen's eyes flickered briefly down the beach. "But Sigeric is a favorite of some of the warriors, those who all along have favored war over negotiation, who want nothing to do with Roman land but to plunder it."

Winnifreya gazed steadily at Dia. "My husband's hopes for settlement are fading—at least, *peaceful* settlement. More and more of the warriors are giving up that hope and seeing it Sigeric's way."

Dia considered the import of her words. "And if Sigeric should somehow sway enough of the warriors to his side and Alaric lose the faith of his men, then I would no longer be valuable as a hostage."

"Exactly."

"So my position is already precarious, and becomes more so the longer negotiations are delayed."

"I see you have a quick grasp of the situation."

"And the delay in negotiations is . . . ?"

"Emperor Honorius."

"Yes, of course."

Winnifreya regarded Dia pityingly. "I find it strange, Galla

Placidia, that your brother has offered us *nothing* for your safe return. Atawulf would move Heaven and Hell to free me if I were held hostage."

Dia looked quickly to sea, toward the crystal-blue horizon, and fixed her gaze there, willing herself not to blink and betray the well of disappointment in her eyes.

"You do not know my brother. His responsibility is the Empire, and the Empire cannot have a weak Emperor. He cannot afford the luxury of capitulation. Besides," she half laughed, "I have difficulty imagining Honorius moving Heaven and Hell." She turned a wistful smile to the queen. "You're fortunate, Winnifreya, to be so sure of your brother. I suspect Heaven and Hell both are dreading Atawulf's arrival."

Winnifreya flung her laughter to the sun. "Oh, I'll be sure to tell Alaric what you said of Atawulf! He'll agree heartily!"

Dia had rarely enjoyed bathing as much as she did that day, whether it was because the bath was so long overdue, or because everything was perfect: the weather was glorious, with a cool breeze, and dazzling white clouds afloat upon an intense blue sky; the water was warm, and the sea sparkled like liquid sapphire. The wet grittiness of the sand and the taste of salt water reminded her of carefree summer days spent at the seashore with her aunts.

She unbraided her hair and let it float free, washed it with peppermint oil, then swam until she was tired. Wading ashore, she slapped more oil on her arms and legs, neck and face, and had Thalia scrape it off with a strigil; then she promptly splashed back into the waves. Eventually she came to sit in the shallows, the tide tickling her feet, the sand filling her hands.

Singledia the Elder arrived with her three young granddaughters, and Singledia the Younger begged to braid Dia's hair, as it was Alfreya's turn to braid their mother's. Dia consented readily.

Usually Dulcie did the braiding, but Dulcie, who arrived on the seashore with a group of freed Germanni, was making a great show of paying no attention to the Imperial Princess, talking and giggling with a group of women and reveling in her free status. Not that Dia cared. That was just like Dulcie, positively overdoing it and making a fool of herself. Dia had no doubt that Dulcie was telling every woman who would listen everything she knew about her former mistress.

Thalia, who had bathed quickly and efficiently, knelt in the water alternately soaking and wringing her mistress's dresses and undergarments. The royal handmaiden had never had to do the work of a laundress, beyond washing out her own few garments, and she felt the work beneath her station. She also noticed Dulcie down the beach, braiding her own hair and enjoying herself with the others.

What was it like, Thalia wondered, to be free? How did it feel? She wished she could ask Dulcie, but what would she say to Dulcie now? She would be embarrassed, and if she would but admit it, Thalia envied Dulcie.

All around Dia the barbarian women bathed, did their washing, and chatted—sometimes in their coarse, incomprehensible Gothic, sometimes in a strange hybrid of Greek and Latin reaped from their wanderings from one end of the Empire to the other. However, Dia made no attempt to converse with any of them beyond the Elder Singledia or the queen and her daughters. An Imperial Princess did not engage in social intercourse with the common class.

Dia noticed with a certain amount of scorn that Queen Winnifreya comported herself in a most undignified manner, chattering away with her subjects as if they were her equals, allowing any of the women to approach her and initiate conversation without waiting for their queen to invite them to speak.

What could one expect, after all, of barbarians?

The Younger Singledia exclaimed over Dia's luxuriously thick hair while she braided it in neat rows. But the girl mourned the short length of the rich brown tresses, for when she tried to weave her creation into a single braid it scarcely brushed past the nape of Dia's neck.

A woman's hair was her glory, she admonished Dia, and

pointed out her mother's hair, which cascaded nearly to her hips. Dia admired Winnifreya's flowing tresses of molten gold to Singledia's satisfaction. Alfreya was braiding it only from the sides, bringing two ropes of sunlit gold together in the back to form one long adorning braid while the rest of the queen's hair fell straight and free.

All the Goths, women and men alike, seemed to grow their hair long, Dia observed aloud. Winnifreya agreed. Women especially felt it a matter of pride to have long hair, and none of them could understand the Roman custom of cutting their hair off simply to make it crimp and curl just so. God created woman's crowning beauty; what made Roman women feel they must improve on it?

Dia laughed, never having thought of it quite that way before, and agreed it did seem rather foolish and vain. But, then, the priests claimed God created women foolish and vain, so it was not surprising that they acted accordingly.

This remark catapulted the Gothic women into a spirited discussion of the foolishness and vanity of their men, which soon became a rapid volley in their own barbaric tongue, leaving Dia at a loss.

She sat on the warm sand, basking in the warm sun, while around her women washed weeks of accumulated sweat from their garments in seawater. Even Winnifreya bent to the task, the Queen of the Goths being accustomed to hard work and the sharing of the load on the long journeys of her people.

It was not until the women were preparing to leave and Thalia was struggling with the full basket of wet clothes, which seemed three times heavier than before, that Singledia the Elder stepped before Dia and blocked her progress up the beach.

"Placidia," the old woman told her in that low, throaty voice, "your maid needs help with your basket."

Dia looked back. Thalia was indeed having trouble carrying the heavy basket.

"Perhaps," suggested Dia, "one of your women would help her."

"All of us have our hands full with our own things. All but you, Princess. You help her."

"I? But I can't carry a basket of laundry."

"And why not?" Singledia's voice cracked like a whip.

"Why . . . it's slave's work . . . you can't possibly expect me to do common slave's work."

"I can, and I do. Everyone does a fair share of the work, even Winnifreya. If my daughter is not above it, neither are you."

Winnifreya had stopped to listen to this exchange. In fact, every woman on the beach stopped to listen.

"You're not serious."

"Oh, I am serious, young lady. If you want that basket of clothes, you'll take hold of one of those handles."

Dia glared at the old crone defiantly, but for the first time in her life Dia did not have unlimited resources at her disposal. She could not replace the garments, and she could not go unclothed.

"What does it matter to you if I carry a basket? Queen Winnifreya, I refuse to take this sort of treatment. Tell her to leave me alone."

The queen shook her head. "I'd sooner tell a bull not to charge, and I'd get the same results. 'Tis simpler to do as she says, Placidia, and not argue, once she's set her mind to meddling. You are meddling somehow, Mother, I know you too well."

Singledia favored her daughter with a mischievous look. "Mind your own business. Well, Placidia, pick up that basket and come along—or do without."

Dia tried to stare the old woman down, but the lucid, sharp eyes were unwavering. Beyond the iron-haired woman Dia saw the three young princesses, their own wet dresses draped over their arms, glance at each other and smile.

Dia set her jaw and glared back at their grandmother. Then

she glanced at Thalia, who stood poised by the heaped basket watching her with intense stillness.

"Oh, very well!" Dia capitulated with less good grace than she might have summoned, but she was too angry at this transparent attempt to humiliate her before all the women. Well, the daughter of Empress Galla and granddaughter of Empress Justina was not so easily humiliated. In a huff she marched to one side of the basket and jerked on the handhold. Thalia, unprepared for this swift capitulation, did not have hold of the other side, and naturally the basket overturned and fine, silken, *wet* garments tumbled onto the sand.

"*Oh, damnation!*" exploded the Most Noble Galla Placidia, which sent the watching Gothic women into shrieks of laughter.

Thalia knelt swiftly to pick up the fallen clothes, but Singledia stopped her with a sharp gesture.

"Galla Placidia, take that childish scowl off your face and pick up your laundry. If you can't handle a simple task any slave can accomplish, how do you expect to handle the difficulties of managing an Empire?"

It was that "you can't handle a simple task" which stuck in her craw. Scarlet-faced, furious, she snatched up the garments and slapped them into the basket. Then she gripped the handle and threw an ominous look at Thalia. This time Thalia was quick to lift the basket with her. Dia glared defiantly at the old woman, but Singledia wordlessly turned on her heel and led the way up the beach.

Princess and slave struggled up the beach with their basket of laundry between them. It was awkward going, trudging along in the sand in fancy sandals, lugging half of a lurching load with one hand, gathering the corner of her fine palla with the other. In her whole life, Dia had never carried a bulky or heavy load. Even as a small child, when such things came naturally, there was always a slave at hand who lifted the burden from her arms and carried it for her.

She was clumsy, too, when it came to coordinating her movements with those of Thalia, so the basket bounced jerkily between them. Thalia, feeling as though she were in a tug-of-war, had to work hard to match her steps with Dia's erratic movements.

"Stop bumping me, Thalia. You're doing that on purpose."

"Oh, no, miss, I'm not."

"I can't make it; my arm's dying. I'm going to drop the basket."

"We could trade sides, miss."

"Trade sides? Oh, of course." Dia dropped her end of the load abruptly, dragging Thalia sideways. "Just look at my hand," moaned Dia, displaying a red indentation across her delicate palm. "It's blistered."

"It doesn't look blistered to me, miss," said Thalia, a trifle impatiently.

"Yes it is. And then it'll be callused, I just know it."

"Yes, yes, I expect it will. And one arm will be longer than the other. The best thing to do is pick up the other side and match them up."

"Thalia, you're poking fun at me."

"This isn't as difficult as you're making it, Mistress Dia."

"You think I'm making a fool of myself, don't you?"

Thalia, to Dia's surprise, winked at her. Annoyed, Dia marched around the basket and gripped the other handle. She said not another word as they trudged into the Gothic camp. She held her head high, her lips firmly set, and she looked neither right nor left until they reached the coach and set the basket down.

With a long-suffering sigh, Dia started to sink to the coach steps, but she halted her descent and stood upright as she saw Singledia approaching.

"Oh, no," Dia murmured. "I wonder what she wants now."

Singledia had a long coil of rope in her hand, which she gave to the guardsman with instructions to string it from the coach to a nearby tree.

Both princess and slave exchanged glances. Then Dia shrugged and picked up a sopping, and now quite gritty, gown and tossed it over the line. Singledia left them to it, looking intolerably smug in Dia's opinion.

"Thalia," she sighed as she helped spread the clothes across the rope, "we've done a poor job of the laundry. Let's pray she doesn't decide we should do our own cooking."

6

The red-tiled roofs of Neapolis glowed crimson in the vivid rays of sunset, hugging the sweeping curve of the splendid blue bay, the smooth, wide waters dark indigo, aquamarine, and sparkling green.

From the rugged promontory on which she stood, Dia could see the whole magnificent Bay of Neapolis laid out before her. The opposite shoreline visible across the expanse of shifting blue was a jagged arm of cliffs jutting into the sea, forming the great curving bay as land stretched out to embrace the sea.

Eastward beyond the city loomed the great mound of Vesuvius, magnificent in its height and breadth, unmoved and undisturbed by the advance of a puny barbarian army. The mountain lay slumbering and still, a thin stream of lazy steam drifting around its peaceful summit.

In the bay floated the beautiful emerald isle of Ischia, glowing green in evening splendor; to the south lay the tiny isle of Capri, rugged and independent, just out of reach of the land's craggy fingertips.

How lovingly Dia remembered that isle, its picturesque little villages and the beautiful palace, the Villa Jovis, where her aunts liked to settle in for the summer. Were her aunts Justa and Grata there now? Perhaps standing atop the hills and squinting across the bay, searching for signs of the Gothic encampment?

Homesickness nearly overwhelmed Placidia, and loneliness. She had not seen Justa and Grata for over two years. Not since Alaric's siege of Rome. Likely her aunts were not on the island at all, but at their country estates in the heart of Italia, but if they were on Capri, at least she knew they would be safe. All the ships in the harbors had set sail at the approach of the barbarian army; the fortunate people with boats or money to buy passage fled to the safety of the sea. The Goths could not reach the island of Capri, even if they captured the harbor city of Neapolis.

Her eyes swept along the curve of the city hugging the nearer shore. Alaric had thus far been unable to breach the inland walls of Neapolis, whose garrison held out valiantly. Dia was glad of that; she cherished happy memories of shopping those gala market streets with her aunts, buying coral and tortoise-shell ornaments, cameos and filigrees, porcelain dolls and little bronze figurines.

But beyond the sun-red roofs of Neapolis Dia could see a glow of another kind—a flickering gloom, plumes of black smoke shrouding the horizon in a broken circle. The Goths wasted no time sitting at the gates of Neapolis; the many cities and towns in the fertile countryside were easy prey. More towns burning, she thought angrily, helplessly. More autumn harvests and winter stores stolen. And anything the Goths could not eat or carry off, they left behind them in flames—fields, orchards, estates, and villages.

Dia's fury and frustration with the destruction of her country tore at her heart and mind. Her heart ached over the desolation wrought upon her homeland, her beloved Italia, the garden of the world. Clenching fists and jaw, she spoke sharply to the man beside her.

"I've seen enough, Rayard. More than enough." She turned, eyes as brooding as the darkling sea, and stalked past her hapless guardsman. He followed soberly, thinking he should not have allowed her a view of the bay, but he had not known the smoke of her burning land would be so visible.

Down the rocky path to the camp, Dia's anger grew and fed on itself with each stumble on the shadowy ground, with each memory of the beautiful towns left in ruins behind the Gothic march, so that by the time she reached the central clearing near her coach she was nearly flying with rage. Rayard had to step lively to keep up with her.

She heard them before she caught sight of them—the Gothic warriors riding back into camp from their day's destruction. They stirred the dust, horses stamping and men shouting to one another, and in their midst rode Alaric and Atawulf, barking orders like two wolves harrying their pack.

Without reflection Dia charged into the midst of the horsemen, intent on at last confronting them face to face. She had been under close guard while the Gothic caravan moved ever southward, and she scarcely ever glimpsed Atawulf. The warriors were busy preying on the countryside, riding in and out of camp, never staying any longer than necessary to drop off their loot.

Startled men reined their mounts aside to let the lone woman pass. She did not halt until she came as near as she dared to the war-horses of Atawulf and Alaric, where she stood her ground defiantly.

"*King* Alaric! *King* of the Goths! You're nothing but a *bandit!* A *renegade* leading a horde of thieves and murderers!"

The King of the Goths stared at his captive as he might stare at one of his recalcitrant daughters. Instead of answering, he aimed a glance of reproach at his brother. Atawulf shrugged and leaned forward in the saddle, his forearm across his thigh, and eyed the angry young woman with rekindled fascination. In the hectic days of riding and raiding he had almost forgotten how beautiful she was; he had almost convinced himself he would never again succumb to the intensity of feeling she evoked in him.

"Answer my charge, King of Jackals!" the princess demanded. "Before God, are you not but a devil and a plague upon decent people? Is this how your brave warriors prove their mettle, by raping the defenseless and robbing the helpless?"

The Gothic horsemen grumbled, and Alaric stiffened, his blue eyes brittle and humorless.

"My warriors would gladly prove their mettle, Princess, if your Roman Legions were brave enough to come and do battle with them."

At that the men laughed and jeered the legions in rude terms. Dia's ears burned as she flushed in humiliation. Alaric was right; where were the legions while the heart of the Empire was pillaged and put to the torch? But she was not to be diverted.

"Does that excuse your savagery?" she snapped. "Or have the Goths never risen above the level of looters and murderers?"

Alaric's sharp-planed face was hard-edged with fury. He roared at her in that terrible battlefield voice which set brave men to quaking. "You will not accost my men with insults and slurs, *Roman!* Roman arrogance and Roman hatred of any nation that does not crawl on its belly to lick the Empire's boots has brought this on you. Let Rome feel the scourge it has laid upon the world since the first Roman slew his brother for dominion over the land."

Dia fought for words, but could as yet find none to refute this attack upon her nation. She lifted her chin defiantly even as her mind whirled to form an attack of her own.

The Bold Wolf sighed hugely, then dismounted and approached the princess. He tried gently to take her arm, but she jerked from his grasp.

Her scathing glance took in his dusty armor—Roman armor—and though with relief she saw no blood upon him, she knew his business had been the taking of towns by force.

"You—you're no better than a . . . a . . ."

"I know—a bandit. Your Royalty, this conversation is better held in private audience with Alaric than in a public shouting match."

"I have not been allowed audience with Alaric, you might have noticed."

Atawulf snickered. "I believe you will have it now." He glanced at his foster brother's glowering face. "You've gained his full attention."

Determined, Dia looked over Atawulf's shoulder and raised her voice imperiously to Alaric. "I demand an audience immediately!"

"Atawulf!" growled the king. "Are you not the man I put in charge of this hostage?"

"Aye," sighed Atawulf.

"Then see if you cannot exercise some little control over her outbursts."

The Bold Wolf reddened as the warriors laughed and cat-called to him. He grabbed Dia roughly by the arm and dragged her away toward the coach, his face flushed with annoyance.

The moment Atawulf's back was safely turned, the King of the Goths dropped all pretense of a scowl and, along with his men, laughed fit to fall off his horse.

"Stop this instant!" Dia said furiously to Atawulf, "I'm not finished with him."

"Oh, aye, you are."

"I will not be ignored!"

"That I grant you. You are *impossible* to ignore."

"What about my audience with Alaric?"

Atawulf stopped short and rounded on her. "What? So he can blame *me* when you badger him to death?"

"I do not badger people!"

In the instant he opened his mouth to reply, Atawulf's glance fell beyond the princess and he spied his brother and king still snickering at his expense. His eyes darted from the grinning figure of Alaric to the determined, stubborn woman defying him with those maddening eyes.

Slowly Atawulf's face broke into a smile that grew larger and brighter. So Alaric liked a clever jest, did he? So did Bold Wolf.

"All right, Your Royal Badgerness, you'll have your audience with Alaric."

Dia regarded his sudden merriment with suspicion.

"When?"

"Tonight. Aye, tonight you dine with the king."

"Oh . . . oh . . ." Surprised by her quick victory, Dia did not quite know what to say. "Well . . . I shall be ready . . . when shall I have Rayard escort me?"

"I will escort you myself. Oh, I wouldn't miss this—your humble self confronting my humble brother."

"Am I supposed to be flattered by your condescension?"

"Why, I thought you'd be most determined to arrive on the arm of no less than the Count of the Domestic Horse."

Dia regarded him scornfully. "If that so-called count *smelled* less like a horse himself, that would be true. You are not fit to escort a laundress direct from the urine vats. If you expect me to arrive on your arm, as you put it, you will first take a bath and change into decent clothes."

"Do I take it you accept my offer? Your charm is so overpowering, Your Royal Graciousness, I am at a loss."

Dia glared at him. "I find it difficult to be gracious to a man who has just come from trampling and burning my own country, killing my own people."

He glowered. "We are doing less killing than you imagine, Princess. We meet little resistance. Our concern now is in the taking of hostages."

"Hostages? Do you mean you are taking Roman citizens?"

"Well-born and rich Roman citizens."

"Of course. For ransom. That is what brigands do, isn't it? Hold wealthy captives for gold."

Atawulf paused, savoring the moment of knowing something she did not. "Gold is not our ransom."

"What then? What is your ransom?"

"Ah, you would like to know, wouldn't you? The answer is not mine to divulge; you'll have to ask Alaric."

"Then I certainly shall. Tonight, you said."

"Aye, tonight. In one hour be ready." With that abrupt command he strode away, snapping a glowering order at Captain Rayard to remain on guard—*if* Rayard could remember that he was supposed to guard the hostage, not escort her about at her royal whim.

Dia watched him leave, wanting to retort that she did not take orders from barbarians, but knowing she would be ready regardless, for she very much wanted this meeting with Alaric. She hurried into her coach, for the daylight hours were short this time of year.

Dusk still lingered, and stars were still slowly creeping into the dark indigo sky, when Atawulf knocked upon the door of the royal coach. Dia, in tiered raiment of green and blue and silver, descended the steps, followed by her handmaiden. In the warm light of a torch held aloft by a Roman slave, Dia noticed with surprise— and some smug gratification—that Atawulf had after all bathed and changed into clean garments. Never mind that those garments were purely barbaric: a leather vest, leather breeches, and thong-bound leggings. Gem-set sword belt, armband, and torque were his only adornments. His flaxen hair was unbraided, still wet, and pulled back with a leather thong.

Mockingly, he offered her his arm, bronze-bare and muscled, but she scorned it, lifting her chin and starting toward the center of the camp. His grin broadened as he swiftly strode into step beside her.

"Not this way, Your Royalty. This." He indicated the opposite direction. "We dine tonight in the villa of this estate we are camped on. The owners appear to have politely left the premises and the stores to their guests."

Silently she turned and accompanied him from the camp. They entered a grey-shadowed grove of olive trees, the slave leading with the torch, Dia and Atawulf walking wordlessly side by side, and Thalia following behind. They emerged upon a path that wound through a shadowy orchard of dry, rattling leaves, passed through a dark hedge, and joined the paved walkways of a sleeping garden.

The villa loomed up in the dark, sitting atop a bare little hill. It was not overly large, and it was new; the walls and portals gleamed brightly as the torchlight danced across their colorful surfaces, scarcely showing the wearing of time. Some poor soul's modest country retreat, thought Dia, overrun by barbarians.

Torches blazed from within the gardens of the peristyle, and a dining room open to the cool fragrance of the courtyard glowed with many lamps. There a small company had gathered for an evening meal. Alaric the king, Queen Winnifreya, Atawulf's brother Wallia, the Gothic bishop, and Priscus Attalus, the Roman Senator turned pretender to the purple.

The company's faces showed their surprise at the arrival of Galla Placidia. The king glowered at his foster brother, who raised hawk-brows in astonished innocence. No one moved to welcome her, until Priscus Attalus rose to his old legs and bowed low. Dia nodded poised acknowledgment toward him before she remembered she cared not how this traitor greeted her. No one else stood, but it was no more than she expected from these rude folk.

"Welcome, Princess Placidia," smiled Winnifreya at last. "We were not expecting you."

"Were you not?" She uncovered her jeweled hair, letting the corner of her silver-stitched palla fall from one bare shoulder and cascade down her back.

The queen's blue eyes held her, unblinking. "No, we have overlooked you, I fear, too long, that you must come unannounced and uninvited." She glanced sidelong at her husband.

"I am invited," Dia told her. "By Atawulf, your brother."

Alaric shifted on his chair, resigned. "Atawulf, who never

thinks to consult his king on any matter, great or small. Well, since you're here, sit, both of you. We're cooling our throats while we await supper."

The Goths, Dia noted, had scorned dining couches and were sitting at the tables in chairs, as was their custom. She refused Atawulf's offer of escort to a chair, and seated herself. She leaned back against the polished wood that curved around, crescent-shaped, to form armrests.

Thalia moved straight to the wine cart and mixed her mistress a goblet of water and wine, which she placed before her mistress; Dia was suddenly glad of her presence. Thalia knew that the Imperial Princess should neither have to wait to be served nor request it, and she saved Dia that indignity. Now Thalia stood quietly behind the princess, to her left, ready to anticipate her every need.

Atawulf, ignoring the frightened motion of a serving slave, poured his own wine undiluted from a pitcher, scorning both the dipper and the water bowl.

Then he boldly plopped down opposite Dia and, stretching his long legs beneath the table, hooked the chair next to her and dragged it closer so that he could prop his leather-bound feet upon its cushioned seat.

Dia bestowed upon him a frosty stare, full of royal pique.

The Bold Wolf chuckled, saluted her with the dripping goblet, and swigged his wine. "Ahhh!" he smacked, wiping his mouth with the back of his hand as the deep red droplets ran down his beard.

Furious, Dia ignored him. If he was bent on being as rude and barbaric as he knew how, then she would treat him with all the disdain he deserved. She lifted her own goblet in a delicate hand.

Queen Winnifreya saw the princess's frosty disapproval of her brother Atawulf, and this she would not countenance. As far as the queen was concerned, her brother could do no wrong, and he was certainly not to be judged lacking by some snub-nosed snippet of a Roman.

"Princess Placidia," Winnifreya told her pointedly, "you are here at the invitation of my brother, and for that reason alone, you have the sufferance of the king."

Dia stiffened in surprise. "I apologize if my presence is unwelcome, Queen Winnifreya. However, I feel it is necessary and proper, as I have been denied my every request for an interview with the king." She regarded Alaric with clear-eyed challenge.

King Alaric met her stare with his own of brilliant blue. His smile was genuine and amiable; Alaric was feeling mellow with the wine and he loved a challenge.

"Never be it said the Goths lack hospitality, Princess," he said, "but I've had other duties more pressing than parrying your insults. Now I am all yours—thrust away, and I will attempt to defend my honor."

Dia's gaze was piercing and steady, her voice even. "You are laughing at me, King Alaric. This is a game to you, is it not? The slaughter of my people, the burning of my country? Pardon me, I pray, if I do not find it so amusing as you do. It is tragic and savage, and I hope against hope that there is some shred of Christian conscience within your Arian faith that I can appeal to."

The smile on Alaric's face hardened into grim anger. "No, this is no game to me. This is war."

"War against whom? The Roman people? They have done nothing to you. This is an invasion, for plunder; and the death of every unarmed man, the rape of every woman, the murder of every child shall be a stone in your soul when you face God's Judgment."

"And how will God judge the Romans' treatment of the Goths?" Alaric retorted sharply. "Why do you not ask yourself that question, Galla Placidia? How will God judge the Empire's treachery?"

"Treachery? Because the Emperor does not open his arms and his Empire to a band of thieves? My brother has seen how you use the trust of emperors."

Alaric waved her words away impatiently. "Your brother is a fool, but I am not! The Goths once believed every Emperor, every promise, and we suffered for our trust. Now we have learned. You are all liars, you Romans."

"And Goths are faithless! You swore to my father you would defend the Empire and uphold his throne. The moment he died you broke faith and plundered and killed. You tried to drive a wedge between East and West; you tried to tear his Empire apart. You made a treacherous pact with Master General Stilicho to divide the Empire between you."

Bold Wolf glowered a warning at Dia across the table, but she ignored him.

"Well?" she demanded. "How do you answer?"

Alaric the king burst into a bout of laughter that startled the villa's slaves so that they nearly dropped the platters they were carrying. Dia glared her indignation.

"I'm so gratified that I amuse you, King of the Goths, but I did not come here to be laughed at by some . . . some *hyena!*"

King Alaric snatched a napkin from the arm of a Roman youth standing at his side and wiped tears of mirth from his eyes. "Hoo! I've fallen in one evening, have I, in your enlightened esteem, from a jackal to a hyena?"

Whereupon he fell into a fit of laughter again.

Dia's face reddened, but more from anger than embarrassment. She thought this barbarian king deserved every beastly name she could think to call him. She glared at Bold Wolf, who was grinning at her.

Queen Winnifreya took matters in hand. She signaled to the slaves to begin serving the first course.

"I believe," said the queen, "that we had best postpone the discussion until we have mastered our tempers and our tongues and are less disposed toward name-calling." Her pale blue gaze rested evenly on Dia.

Dia accepted this criticism with less grace than she ought, meeting Winnifreya's gaze with the frosty stare of royal indifference she had learned so well from Serena. But Winnifreya merely smiled knowingly and raised her cup to Dia.

Silence reigned as pigeon soup and stuffed eggs were served. The king slurped hot soup directly from the bowl and licked his lips with satisfaction.

"Now that you've had your say, Princess . . ."

"I have not. The audience is not over."

"The audience is over when I say it is over!"

Both pairs of eyes blazed with myriad flecks of light from the oil lamps. Alaric sighed.

"For now, let us call a truce—temporary only, do not worry, Princess—so that we may at least digest our dinner. Conversation with you is giving me heartburn." He put a hand to his chest and belched loudly.

If he meant to offend Dia, he miscalculated. She smiled pleasantly, delighted to cause him heartburn or any other discomfort.

"Very well. Truce—until after dinner." She sipped her soup daintily from a long-handled silver spoon.

Winnifreya spoke to set the conversation on a safe track. "Placidia, I don't know if you've met our younger brother, Wallia—Atawulf's brother and mine. He's one of our finest war leaders." She nodded toward a youthful warrior, scarcely older than Placidia herself, a smiling man who obviously shared their bloodline.

He saluted the princess with his cup. "Your Royalty, I'm honored. I've long admired your beauty from afar, where Atawulf has made sure I've stayed."

She acknowledged him with a slight nod. "General Wallia."

At that Atawulf snorted. Wallia's eyes widened and he scrambled to his feet.

"General, you say. Princess, I am at your service evermore." Then for the first time one of the Goths actually bowed to Dia. She took an immediate liking to Wallia.

"General Swell-Head is more like it," Atawulf told Dia.

"He's been trying to get everyone to call him 'General' for months."

"Perhaps he wears his title with more pride than you do, *Count* Atawulf. Is it of no consequence to you?"

" 'Tis a Roman title."

"Yet you took it. Stole it, rather."

"A political expediency," said Atawulf, glancing good-naturedly toward the ex-pretender to the purple, Priscus Attalus. "I prefer to be a simple Gothic warrior. The *best* Gothic warrior, mind you, but—"

Now Wallia snickered loudly into his cup. "But the *simplest!*" he finished for his brother.

Atawulf threw an egg at him, striking him aside the head, but Wallia merely laughed louder. Dia realized he was too deep in his cups to care. She looked to Queen Winnifreya, who seemed unaffected by her brothers' rude behavior. In fact, the queen was sending the Roman youth to the cart for another cup of wine.

Winnifreya noticed Dia's glance. "We are very informal here, Placidia, as you have observed. Does Roman royalty never let down its hair?"

"Not in quite the same fashion," said Dia.

Winnifreya laughed and the silken strands of her long golden hair draped across her sun-brown arms. Her tunic was sleeveless, and the shapely curves of her upper arms were encircled with bands of gem-set gold.

"I imagine a Roman supper is quite stuffy. You really must have a little more wine, Placidia, and enjoy the company. You've met our bishop, I believe—Bishop Sigesarius."

The bishop inclined his head. He was elderly and weathered, in travel-worn brown robes; grey hair hung in wisps about his furrowed face.

"He introduced himself to me," Dia acknowledged.

"Prematurely perhaps, nobilissima," said the bishop. "Now that you have spent more time in our company, I extend the invitation again. My door is always open—or, rather I should say, my tent flap—should you feel the need for spiritual comfort."

Dia regarded him gravely. "I appreciate your kind offer, Father. I hope you understand my position; as a daughter of the True Church, I cannot in good conscience seek spiritual counsel from an Arian bishop."

"Come, come," burst in Priscus Attalus. "Let's have no religious debates, please, nobilissima, Bishop."

Dia swallowed the last of her watered wine and set down the empty cup. She regarded the intruder coolly. "Then what shall we debate, Attalus? Patriotism? Treason?"

Bold Wolf intercepted her cup, whisking it from a startled Thalia's fingers. "Allow me, Your Royalty."

The former Senator flushed. "I am not a traitor, nobilissima, no matter what you believe."

"What do you call this, if not treachery? Throwing in your lot with barbarians?"

"A reasonable response to an unfortunate—and unnecessary—crisis. *Someone* had to act for the safety of the people of Rome, to break the siege and halt the starvation. The Emperor abandoned them to their fate."

"And your response was to usurp the throne and rule as the puppet of barbarians."

"At least there would be rule," snapped Attalus. "No act of mine could be worse than your brother's incompetence."

"How dare you call your Emperor incompetent!"

"How dare I not, if I care for Rome!"

King Alaric laughed aloud. "Priscus cared more for Rome than for the throne, Princess. The old fool balked me on so many matters I had to demote him."

Bold Wolf set the refilled goblet at Dia's hand. Serving slaves began removing bowls and replacing them with platters of pickled fishes and snails and turbot in cream sauce, part of the villa's preserved stores.

So the King of the Goths was on a first-name basis with Priscus Attalus, Dia thought indignantly. She swallowed a mouthful of wine and nearly choked on its overpowering sweetness. It was unwatered.

"Are you hoping to make me drunk?" she accused Atawulf.

Bold Wolf propped his feet on the table. "That might be interesting." He rolled his own goblet between his palms.

"I am never drunk," she assured him, sipping gingerly from the silver rim.

"Afraid your protocol will slip, Your Correctness?"

"Afraid? I should say not. But I'm sure I would find the experience humiliating and undignified."

Atawulf raised both blond eyebrows in mock surprise. "You? Undignified?"

Dia shot him an end-of-her-patience look and stabbed at a creamed snail with the pointed end of her spoon. To her annoyance, the snail slipped across the platter and onto the table. Atawulf skewered it expertly and slurped it down.

"Your table manners are atrocious," she said.

"You'd be disappointed if they weren't."

"I refuse to speculate on what you mean by that remark."

The Bold Wolf merely smirked at her behind his beard.

Winnifreya clucked at them reprovingly from the end of the table.

Their startled gazes met her amused expression. Suddenly Dia felt very foolish. Appalled that she had quite forgotten herself and bickered like a . . . a housemaid with this barbarian, she glanced guiltily at him, only to meet his mischievous grin. Dia glared and snatched up her winecup. How did he always manage to do this to her?

She had forgotten, of course, that the wine was unwatered, and her angry swallow brought surprise to her eyes, followed by a gasping cough and choking tears. To her embarrassment, Atawulf attempted to stretch across the table and pound her on the back, but she shoved his arm away and wrenched her chair back to avoid his reach. The chair caught on the leg of another and toppled backward, carrying her over with it, and she sprawled abruptly and picturesquely upon the tiled floor.

Atawulf leaned across the table in alarm and discovered her in a decidedly scenic position. His jaw worked. Her furious glare dared him to laugh.

"Well, Your Royalty," he drawled happily, "I see you've landed on your dignity. And I was afraid you were going to disappoint me."

"Oh!"

Dia struggled to her feet. Thalia hastily straightened her mistress's chair, but could not look at Placidia. Dia did not miss the quirky smile Thalia's bent head tried to conceal behind the veil of black hair. Even her maid was laughing at her. What a spectacle she must have made of herself.

At this thought, Dia leaned upon the table and dropped her head into her arms, utterly defeated by the evening's debacle. Her neck flushing crimson, she suddenly raised her head and sat upright, tears streaming from her eyes as she sat helplessly laughing.

Gasping for air, she wiped the tears away with her fine palla. Atawulf beamed at her. He had never seen any woman look so beautiful and vibrant and foolish all in one moment.

"Oh, mercy, mercy!" she sighed, and reached for the wine goblet again. This time, with a high-spirited glance toward Atawulf, she sipped the unwatered wine with care.

Everyone was in high spirits by now. Wallia swayed to his feet and toasted the Imperial Princess.

"To Her Royalty! We never knew you were such a good sport—or so graceful!"

"Aye!" chimed in King Alaric, clambering to his feet also. "Had I known you were so entertaining, Princess, I would have invited you to dinner every evening."

Winnifreya joined in, eyes sparkling, raising her cup high

above her head. "Placidia, Placidia, I beg your pardon for ever thinking you were stuffy. I've not laughed so hard in ages. I thank you."

Bold Wolf rose to his feet, his dark blue eyes dancing in the lamplight. He paused, drinking in the sight of her, the color of her deep-sea eyes, the loosened strands of honey-brown hair curling down her flushed cheeks and neck, the gentle, unguarded smile on her moist lips, and he could think of nothing to say. His eyes held hers fast for a space of breathless heartbeats, then he raised his cup silently, drained it, and sat down.

Flustered, freed from his compelling gaze, Dia fingered the silver stem of her goblet and avoided looking at him. The intense look in his deep indigo eyes quite unnerved her, and why did her heart race and skip so wildly?

Winnifreya and Alaric exchanged keen glances.

Dinner continued merrily after the laughter, and the company was feeling quite mellow with the wine. Dia, too, sipping strong, spicy libations, felt a cozy warmth spread throughout her limbs, and the lamplight seemed a peaceful, golden glow of goodwill. She smiled blissfully.

While waiting for dessert, King Alaric accepted another drink from the Roman youth at his elbow and waved a hand magnanimously toward Dia.

"Well, Princess, you had more matters to discuss with me, I believe. Now is the time—I am in an excellent mood to discuss anything you please."

Dia blinked at him. What had she meant to say to the King of the Goths? She took several seconds to gather her thoughts.

"Ah, yes," she began in honey-coated tones. She swallowed against the sweet fuzziness in her throat and began again, this time more firmly.

"Hostages. I came to speak to you about the hostages you are taking. Wealthy, noble-born citizens. It is not to be borne." She frowned, aware that her choice of words was repetitious. Pushing away the nearly empty cup, she sat up straighter in the chair and firmly focused her wandering mind.

"These are wealthy people you are taking, women and children among them. I assume you have some ransom in mind."

Alaric grinned hugely. "Possibly."

"What is your ransom?"

"You'd be surprised."

"Do you really think my brother will give you what you want just because you hold more hostages?"

"No. I expect your brother will give me nothing. If he would not ransom all of Rome or even his own sister, then he will surely not ransom a lot of blue-blooded merchants."

"Then what do you hope to gain?"

Alaric chewed his lip and stared at her. "Why this sudden concern over hostages, Your Royalty? I didn't see you expressing concern in Rome when we took all the slaves we wanted."

"Those were slaves; these are citizens."

"*Rich, noble* citizens."

"Yes. There is a great difference."

"I see. The greater the personage, the greater the crime."

"By Roman law, yes, that's true," Dia replied thoughtfully.

Alaric waved toward the Roman youth at his side. The young boy, perhaps fourteen years old, stepped forth. He bowed proudly. His bold brown eyes met those of the Imperial Princess with childlike fascination and manlike seriousness. A momentous occasion in his young life, this, being presented to the Most Noble Princess Galla Placidia.

"This young man, son of one of your most valiant generals, Gaudentius, and one of your wealthiest noblewomen, was given me as hostage by Emperor Honorius himself. Now, if I were a vengeful man, your brother's attack while we were engaged in treaty negotiations would give me every right to have this boy executed. Do you agree?"

Dia was stunned. "Honorius gave you hostages and then broke the truce?"

Alaric's waiting silence answered her.

"Yes," she conceded reluctantly, "you have the right. But it would be monstrous—to kill this boy who is innocent of any act of my brother's."

"Any more monstrous than your brother throwing him to the lions, as it were? A sacrificial lamb? He was twelve years old when he came to me."

Dia shuddered and looked at the boy, strong-limbed, straight-backed, sunny-eyed. "Yet, you have taken good care of him."

Alaric nodded. "I'm fond of Aetius. I knew his father well, in fact. We were rival captains in the legions. General Gaudentius was of half-Germanni blood himself—did you know that?—which makes his son our distant cousin."

"No, I didn't know that."

"I could no more kill Aetius than my own flesh and blood, and it would not matter to the Emperor if I did. Your precious Romans are safer with me, Princess, than with your brother."

Dia shook her head. "You've killed many Romans, King Alaric."

"None of them hostages."

She regarded him for a long moment. "I sincerely hope that remains your policy in the future."

Alaric laughed loudly. "I don't know, Galla Placidia. You try my patience sometimes. I could make an exception." His tone was one of good-natured jest, not meant to be threatening, and he was pleased that Placidia had the good sense to take it as such. The King of the Goths could not bear a humorless wit in man or woman.

Dia took a cautious sip of Herculean-strength wine with an I'm-on-to-you glance at Atawulf, for it was he who had again refilled her cup. Bold Wolf was enjoying himself immensely. He suspected the Imperial Princess had not finished with Alaric, and he looked forward to a further sharpening of wits between her and his foster brother.

She did not disappoint him. "Still, Alaric," she said, "if I may be so informal, I do not see that you stand to gain anything by taking hostages. Why use a strategy that gives you no advantage, if strategy it is? As far as I can ascertain, you have no plan of campaign at all. You are simply fleeing south into the toe of Italia, where you must eventually turn about and retreat."

"We are not *fleeing,* Princess. If you perceive no strategy, that is forgivable. You have less experience in campaigns than I do."

"But why burn the land, all the crops, behind you if not to slow pursuit?"

"I'm a cautious man. There might have been pursuit; in fact, there *should* have been. But the truth is, no legions are following us. My scouts report no legions on the move in Italia at all."

"There!" Dia said triumphantly. "My brother knows you will have no choice but to return up the peninsula, and he awaits your return, when your men are tired and hungry and his rested and well-fed."

Alaric shook his head. "No, the Emperor sits in Ravenna surrounded by two legions, which he will not let march one mile away lest the invaders in Gaul break through the Alps and catch him unguarded. He protects his own sacred person and cares nothing for the suffering of the rest of the country—or for the fate of his sister."

That stung. Dia's green eyes glittered. "My brother must be sorely besieged."

"He is not. His commander in Gaul has the invaders themselves under siege, as I hear it. The truth is, Princess, your brother is a coward."

"Not true!" she denied. "There must be good reason . . ."

"What other reason? Tell me, would your father—would Theodosius—be hiding behind his legions in Ravenna? And what would Theodosius think of his son's magnificent lack of action?"

Dia sank back in her chair and regarded Alaric gravely. "My father . . . my father never hid from battle, never thought of his own safety in his life."

Alaric nodded his sincere acknowledgment of that truth.

"You see, when you consider what old Theo would have done, your brother's *strategy* is nothing but indifference and self-interest."

Atawulf felt a stab of pity for the young woman sitting across from him. She dejectedly turned her silver-stemmed goblet around and around on the tabletop. Dessert was served and ignored. The company sat silent and somber.

Dia at last lifted her cup and drank deliberate, deep swallows. Then she slammed the goblet onto the table, splashing wine like blood across her hand.

"Oh, Holy Mother, would that I were a man!"

Bold Wolf, cup poised halfway to his mouth, could only think what a tragedy that would be.

"If I were Emperor," Dia told Alaric vehemently, "you would never have gotten this far! I would have destroyed your army the first time you camped before the gates of Rome! I would have ridden at the head of the legions and scattered you like vermin!"

Their stunned silence rang in Dia's ears, but she was feeling reckless and tragic and was beyond caring that she had shocked, quite possibly enraged, her captors. She stared unflinchingly at the King of the Goths.

He stared back, equally unflinching. Finally Alaric spoke, his tone surprisingly mild. "We are fortunate that you do not wear the purple, Galla Placidia."

"Very fortunate."

"I suspect that you would make a far better Emperor than your brother. And a more formidable adversary." He shook his head almost with regret. "Such a war we would have fought."

"Yes," agreed Dia, with equal regret. She nodded at the visions she saw deep within her cup. "I would challenge you to single combat and slay you with a mighty stroke and save my people, my country, my Empire."

"I would fight ferociously," he said, sharing her wine-haloed vision. "You might lose."

"Then I would die honorably, in battle, a warrior."

Bold Wolf, listening, nodded approval. "No better way to die," he murmured.

Queen Winnifreya shifted impatiently in her chair. "Are you all going maudlin on me? I, for one, am disappointed in you, Galla Placidia. I would hope for a wiser solution from the daughter of Theodosius."

"Such as . . . ?"

"A wise Emperor would have avoided the crisis altogether by dealing fairly and honestly with us in the first place. You could have made us a fair treaty."

"You mean bow to your threats?"

"No, I mean, we would be an asset to the Empire as a settled nation—"

"*Sovereign* nation, do I take it?"

"Of course. Our own laws, our own king, yet loyal to the Emperor. We would defend the borders; we could be now defending the throne from the usurpers in Gaul."

"You had your chance. The Goths deserted the army after my father died."

"Even your father turned on us in the end. We had even less chance of fair treatment after he died."

"Oh? Not even from your friend Master General Stilicho?"

Now Winnifreya laughed. The queen, as deep in revelry as the warriors, had a laugh throaty and sensuous.

"Oh, really, Placidia! Do you honestly believe that we were in league with Stilicho and his wife, Serena?"

"Honorius had reason to believe it."

"*Honorius!*" The outburst came from Bold Wolf. His blue eyes glittered at Dia, and a sneer twisted his lips. "Honorius is worse than incompetent, worse than a fool. He is *stupid!* He cut his own throat when he assassinated Stilicho."

Dia was caught off-guard by the contempt with which Atawulf spoke of her brother. What if it were true? If there was no conspiracy? Oh, Holy Mother of God! *Cousin Stilicho!*

Her defense of her brother was weakened by doubt, her voice small and wavering. "There was evidence—you made pacts with him."

"Of course we made pacts with him!" retorted Atawulf. "We made pacts with him because we had to. Stilicho was the only thing standing between us and the Western Empire. Stilicho was the only general who knew how to lead an army, the only one who could hold us back—and your brother had him beheaded!" Words were not enough. Atawulf spat in disgust.

Dia stared at him, but her eyes, pale and pain-glazed, were unseeing. She was seeing Stilicho, dear Cousin Stilicho, who had been loyal to her father, even after his death—even supporting his incompetent, foolish, *stupid,* ungrateful son on the Imperial Throne. Cousin Stilicho, who had surrendered to the clemency of her brother and been beheaded on the spot for his loyalty.

Shuddering, she closed her eyes, unwilling to face the truth, unable to deny it. Tears leaked from beneath the dark veils of her lashes and trickled in hot streams down her cheeks.

The company was so surprised they came perilously close to sober. The king narrowly staved off disaster by swaying to his feet and raising his cup to the departed.

"To Stilicho!" he said effusively. "We fought as brothers-in-arms, once upon a time. The best man to stand beside shoulder-to-shoulder, and the fiercest enemy shield-to-shield. I admired the general greatly, almost as much as he admired me." Alaric rolled his eyes to Heaven, his voice choked with sentiment. "Ah, Stilicho, I miss you. Who shall be my match now? And to think, you died like a dog."

"Aye, aye," slurred the company, raising their cups and drinking to the dead.

Now even Priscus Attalus rose slowly to his feet. "To Master General Stilicho!" he cried. "Defender of Rome!" The old statesman turned confidentially to King Alaric. "He rebuilt the walls, you know, which held so long against you."

Alaric nodded gravely and drank again to Stilicho.

Dia's tears increased to torrents upon hearing these testaments to her kinsman's loyalty. Cradling her head in her hands, she sobbed brokenly. Thalia, knowing how real Dia's pain was at this moment, knelt by her side to comfort her, laying a gentle arm across her mistress's quivering shoulders. Winnifreya, overcome, left her chair and rushed forward, flinging her arms around both princess and handmaiden.

Queen Winnifreya was at her most maudlin. She squeezed them together affectionately in a powerful, if drunken, embrace. Thank goodness, Thalia thought wryly, she'll not likely remember this in the morning.

Atawulf stumbled to his feet, affected deeply by the women's emotional outpouring. His voice was thick with feeling.

"To Stilicho! A true barbarian!"

"Aye!" chorused all the men except Wallia, who had slid quietly to the floor and now lay snoring under the table.

Dia raised her head abruptly, bumping the queen's nose; the queen staggered backward with a gasp and felt gingerly to see if her nose was flattened.

Glaring at Atawulf defiantly through reddened and weepy eyes, Dia shook Thalia off and stood—too quickly. The colorful dining room danced crazily for a moment, and she leaned a hand upon the table until the spinning stopped. She managed to right herself and lift her own winecup.

"To Cousin Stilicho! A true *Roman!*"

The company cheerfully agreed.

Dia remained standing and sniffed tearfully. "I always felt in my heart he was innocent," she told them, defending her part. "Honorius had him killed before I even knew he was charged."

"I, too," broke in Priscus Attalus, "I never believed it of Stilicho."

Dia blinked at him. "You? It was you who brought me that wretched petition!"

"*You* signed it," Attalus was quick to point out.

"*You* wanted it signed!"

The former Prefect shrugged. "So did you, nobilissima," he reminded her bluntly.

Dia stared at him in shock, then blindly she sat down, nearly missing the chair, which Thalia hastily maneuvered beneath her.

"What petition?" wondered Atawulf.

"Isn't it obvious?" said Queen Winnifreya, who was none too pleased with the Imperial Princess at this moment. "The petition condemning Stilicho's wife to death. For treason." She sat with stiffened spine, dabbed at her nose with a napkin wetted in wine, and addressed Dia accusingly. "If you didn't believe Stilicho was guilty of conspiracy, then how is it you believed it of Serena?"

"I . . . I couldn't be sure . . . but it stood to reason that Honorius *must* have evidence against Stilicho . . . so it was possible that Serena . . ." Dia's excuses trailed off into silence, for she knew them for what they were. She never really believed Serena guilty of treason—she *hated* Serena and wanted revenge for everything Serena had ever done to her. Then suddenly that petition . . .

Incredibly, Priscus Attalus rose to her defense. "What else should she believe? The Senate had condemned Serena unanimously."

Atawulf's eyes on Dia glittered like an icy sea. "So you cold-bloodedly signed her death warrant. Your own kinswoman. What you did was no different, no better, than what your brother did to Stilicho."

No! Dia wanted to scream at him. *It was different! You didn't know her! How cruel and hateful she was, and what she did to people!* But the Imperial Princess of Rome could not admit those things. To act out of passion and not reason was disgraceful in one of royal blood. She had always been admonished that the heart should never rule the head. *And who taught me that?* she realized with bitter irony. *Serena.*

The Bold Wolf saw the bitter smile that fleetingly touched those sensuous lips, and he shuddered inwardly. What sort of woman was Galla Placidia truly? Had he been fooled entirely by that lovely face, that childlike innocence, and those exquisitely guileless eyes?

A murder of passion he could understand; it was part of a warrior's honor—the oath of vengeance sworn in blood. But the cold and calculated execution of close kindred, especially of the woman who had raised her from childhood—this was beyond the bounds of honor. This was . . . *Roman!* Father in Heaven, how could he forget? She was a Roman Imperial, twice royal, and twice infected with all their vices, perfidy, and deceit.

Dia was quick to catch the look of condemnation in his eyes, and the guilt which had been her burden for so long raised its ugly head and rose to its own defense. She met his gaze coldly, calling up all her court training, and her eyes were as hard as blue topaz.

"It was the will of the people," she told him with impenetrable finality, "and the will of the Senate—and mine also. I signed the petition because I believed it to be in the best interest of Rome. My actions are not subject to your approval. God will be my judge, Atawulf—not you."

Their eyes clashed, smoldering blue and adamant aquamarine, in stubborn challenge.

Bishop Sigesarius nodded and waved an arm in enthusiastic, intoxicated agreement. "The very truth, Princess Placidia, eloquently put. We, being merely human, as you are, must presume that you acted with the best intentions."

Atawulf, feeling he was being chastised by the bishop, flung one last glare at the woman and thrust himself from the table.

Dia, feeling that the bishop spoke directly to her guilty secret, pushed back her chair also.

To their amazement and dismay, Dia and Atawulf unexpectedly found themselves both standing, facing each other across the table. For a long space, no one moved, no one spoke, all eyes on the two of them.

Bishop Sigesarius leaned over toward Priscus Attalus to murmur bemusedly in his ear. "What did I say?"

Priscus Attalus shrugged. "Who knows? Youngsters are so hot-headed." *Especially, he refrained from adding, youngsters so obviously besotted with each other as these two.*

"I . . . it's getting late," stammered Dia. "I would like to leave now." She turned to Winnifreya. "It's been a lovely evening, but . . . I believe I've had a little too much wine." Then to Alaric: "Thank you for the audience. It was very . . . enlightening. I . . ." Her eyes touched on Atawulf, then slipped away, avoiding him. She swallowed hard and went on more firmly. "Good-night. Thalia . . ."

Thalia stepped quietly forward and settled Dia's light, shimmery palla across her shoulders and expertly draped its soft folds over her jewel-pinned hair.

Atawulf's breath lodged in his throat. He had never known a woman so painfully desirable, nor one he less wished to affect him so.

The king and queen bid Dia a mellifluous good-night, and she departed the dining hall with a slow dignity, slow because she had to tread carefully across the mosaicked floor. Emerging into the open space of the peristyle, she breathed thankfully the cool night air, which cleared her head.

Atawulf dropped heavily into his chair, ignoring the fact that Alaric looked at him expectantly.

"Go with her," said his foster brother.

Atawulf shook his head, reached for his winecup, which he found empty.

"You know better than to let her wander about alone, Atawulf."

"Send someone else."

"You brought her here, if you remember, and not at my request. She's your charge, brother, and if she never makes it back to camp, don't think I won't hold you responsible."

"Oh, hell, Alaric! What do you think is going to happen between here and camp?"

"She might escape. I wouldn't be surprised."

"Good riddance."

"Atawulf," growled the king, "that is a command."

Atawulf glared hard at his foster brother. Finally he shoved to his feet. "All right, I'm going."

Atawulf dashed into the middle of the peristyle and looked about. Its torch-thrown shadows revealed nothing but carefully trimmed trees and bushes. He could see straight through the tablinum into the atrium, and into the vestibulum; she could not possibly have left the villa so quickly unless she ran—or was hiding.

Atawulf pounced upon a passing slave, a balding man replacing burned-out torches in the peristyle.

"The princess! Where did she go?"

Staring at the barbarian as if he were a madman, the slave pointed to a lighted opening off the entrance to the garden. "To the latrine, master."

"Is there another door? Another exit from the latrine?"

"No, no other," said the man. "She must come out this way."

Atawulf relaxed. "Good. I'll wait." The barbarian made use of the time, and of the azaleas, to relieve himself of the wine he had consumed, much to the disgust of the slave, who in fact tended those azaleas with meticulous care. He hoped the invaders would be gone in the morning.

At last Dia emerged from the latrine, accompanied by her handmaiden.

"Sick, Your Royalty?"

She started, hearing his voice and glimpsing his form in the shadows. Her heart beat wildly, which she attributed, with some annoyance, to finding him lurking about in the bushes like some assassin.

"No, I am not sick. I feel perfectly fine, thank you." She paused to confront him. "Am I allowed no privacy whatsoever, that you must accompany me even to the latrine? Do you not wish to enter within and see that I did my business properly?"

He grinned at her. "Your Royalty, I'm sure your business is the same as everyone else's. I'm here to escort you back to camp. Alaric thought you might lose your way in the dark."

"Escape, don't you mean?"

"That did cross his mind."

"But not yours?"

"Never."

"Never? Do you imagine I am afraid to escape?"

"No, but I know you better than you think, Your Royalty. You're dying to know where we're going and why, and what we'll do when we get there. I'll bet the last thing you want to do right now is go back to court and idle away your days with all that precious protocol and dull routine."

Dia stared at him, speechless. She wanted to deny that he knew anything about her whatsoever and that he was absolutely wrong—the very idea!

Yet something in his words tugged at her conscience. Of course she would go home this very minute, given the opportunity. This was not her life, this homeless wandering, this primitive existence. But when she returned to that comfortable world of protocol and dull, yes, *dull* routine, she would remember moments of this journey as the most vivid, alive moments of her life. And not the least of those vivid memories would be this rough blond warrior grinning at her.

Her pulse leapt as she looked into the depths of those deep blue eyes, and she felt a slow flush heating her face. She tore her gaze away and stepped past him.

"Ridiculous," she said. "I have absolutely no interest in the Goths, present or future, beyond a hope that you will recognize your folly, release me, and depart the Empire forever. If you imagine otherwise, then you must be drunk."

"Aye, I must be," muttered Atawulf, staring after her, noting the graceful swaying contours of her silken gown as she walked away.

He started into the atrium after her and nearly collided with Thalia. The Greek slave stopped short and bestowed upon him a swiftly penetrating stare, a look in those jet eyes of both inquiry and warning. Then the slave stepped back to let him pass ahead of her. His warrior's stride quickly caught up with the princess and he fell into place alongside her, neither hindering her nor offering his arm; he knew better.

She afforded him one sidelong glance, having fully expected him, of course, for she had no more intention of walking back alone in the dark than he had of allowing her. With Atawulf, she felt protected, for who would accost the Bold Wolf?

Strange, she realized suddenly, looking at the barbarian beside her as they emerged into the silvery night, but she felt perfectly safe with Atawulf. Why did that thought surprise her and bring her to a standstill upon the villa steps?

The half-moon rode high, and as Atawulf turned his head to look at her, his hair glimmered silver-white in the streaming moonlight, and his eyes danced with dark and light like stars at midnight.

Dia caught her breath. Had she never noticed how beautiful he was?

A smile flashed in the pale silver of his beard.

"A moonlight walk, Princess?"

"Alone? With you?"

"We have your guardian angel here." He swept a hand toward Thalia, who had come up silently behind them. "A night like this just begs to be walked in."

Dia laughed softly. "Yes, it does." She inhaled the fresh air, fragrant with life, and turned her face to the moon, whose bright half-disk flooded the sky with gossamer light, outshining the star-strewn heavens.

Across the grey lawn shimmered a path of white stone, spanning the pale night like a radiant ribbon of light, beckoning.

Drawn, they stepped off the portico together and walked the moonpath, crossing the grassy expanse that sloped down to the gardens. The moon-frosted path became a patterned web of walkways shimmering between dark flowerbeds and mysterious clumps of shrubbery. Unhurriedly they made their way across the garden on paths of moonlight.

"Peace," murmured Atawulf, filling his soul with the night.

"What?"

"Peace. This is peace. At times something reminds me what peace is like, and I try to make it a part of me, so that I can remember it . . . later."

"You want peace so much?"

"Sometimes my heart aches for it."

Dia halted suddenly and turned to face him. "I had no idea."

"What? That a savage beast like me might prefer peace?"

"No, that a *Goth* might."

"You believe Goths wish to be eternally at war? Do you think we love this life—always on the move, living on what we can plunder, having nowhere to settle?"

"Well, I assumed . . . you *seem* to love it. If you hate war so much, why do you pursue it? Why do you follow Alaric?"

Atawulf snorted rudely. "You think Alaric prefers war?"

"I do. And he makes it no secret that he hates Romans."

"He has good reason."

"As Romans have good reason to hate him. Why could not you Goths just have stayed on the other side of the Danubius if you despise the Empire so much?"

Atawulf's voice was raw. *"Would to God that we had!"*

Dia, taken aback by the anger and pain in his outcry, could not find words that would not seem flippant or callous. She peered searchingly at him in the moonlight, trying to read his face.

"Why?" she finally said, her voice almost a whisper. She felt a strange ache in her own heart, as though she had lost something precious.

"Why are we enemies, Atawulf?"

She heard his sharp intake of breath, then the heavy sigh as he slowly expelled it.

"You know why. It began before we were born. The stupid thing is, we were *willing!*" Savagely he turned and struck his palm to his fist. "The Goths were *willing* to live peacefully in the Empire. It would have been a good alliance. Then the Romans betrayed us."

Atawulf turned his eyes to the moon, as though he saw the past written there. "I was not yet born, but Alaric was—Alaric remembers. He remembers how hungry he was, and he remembers his mother trading the use of her body to a Roman officer for meat, and he remembers his mother dying in vomit and agony of the diseased meat they gave her—*dog* meat. Alaric was six years old."

Atawulf's jaw muscles bunched tightly. "Alaric nearly died, too. My mother nursed him through it, but nothing could touch his grief."

Dia bowed her head. No, nothing could touch the grief of a child so young losing a mother. She fingered the slender chain on the gold locket she wore next to her bosom.

"Our fathers," Atawulf said hoarsely, pausing to clear his throat, "our fathers, Alaric's and mine—though I was not yet born—were taken away with the warriors. The Romans had separated them from the women and children and guarded them with the legions. In exchange for food, the Romans demanded the children as hostages. And our fathers had no choice. Most of their weapons had been seized during the river crossing.

"Winnifreya was but a nursling, but Alaric was six years old, just the age Romans liked to take them. So Alaric went to the Romans.

"He doesn't speak much of that time, except to say he was treated with contempt. You Romans believe we are savages and that somehow your cruelties are more civilized than ours. For the noble cause of *civilization,* Alaric was stripped of his people, his language, his customs, and told he was dirty, ignorant, savage, little better than an animal. Oh, he learned, all right; he learned to speak and act Roman, and he learned to respect the ruthless power of Rome almost as much as he hated it."

Atawulf swallowed hard. "It was a terrible time for Alaric. Goths are taught to bow to no one; we are taught to stand tall, stand proud. And Romans tried to make him despise his own people, despise himself, and worship them. But Alaric was not so easily beaten. He has never forgotten those days of keeping silent, keeping still, while they scorned his people, his very blood.

"Eventually, the warriors broke free of the Empire's armies and took food and weapons by force. They freed the captive children, as many as could be found. Alaric was lucky. He and several older boys being 'civilized' were housed together; they escaped over the wall at night, stole horses, and rode to freedom.

"Other Gothic captives were not so lucky. Romans massacred them by the thousands. It was too late for them when we finally defeated the legions at Adrianople.

"Alaric's father fell in that battle, routing the Roman cavalry, and Alaric was left an orphan. My father, Sigiswulf, took him as his foster son. I was born that year, and I've always had Alaric to look to, my older brother."

He turned to her defiantly. "You accuse Alaric of being a brigand, a marauder, a savage destroying your precious *civilization*. Well, the Goths have reason to hate Rome, and Alaric no less than any."

Whatever retort he expected, she surprised him, her eyes soft in the moonlight, with gentle words that found the unspoken in his heart.

"You love Alaric very much."

Atawulf's widened eyes bared his soul for a moment, revealing the depth of his love for his splendid, boastful, courageous foster brother. Abruptly he turned the open windows of his eyes again to the half-dark moon.

"Aye. Aye, I do."

Dia, spellbound by his fair face, his chiseled, crag-rough features now a silvery gold color of moonlight, felt a strange yearning in her breast. *Oh, to see eyes so full and bright with me as Atawulf's are with Alaric. What joy to be loved so much—loved by the Bold Wolf.*

Disquieted by her wayward imagination, Dia spun abruptly and walked along the path.

"We should be getting back now." Her voice sounded small and uncertain.

"Why?" He strode beside her, through the dark tunnel of the hedge. They emerged beneath the sleeping orchard, an intricate canopy of black velvet and silver lace.

"Why?" he repeated.

"It's . . . late."

" 'Tis early yet."

"Well, it's . . ." She could think of no reason she could admit to.

"Improper?" he teased.

"Yes . . . improper," she breathed. "Terribly improper."

His chuckle was a disbelieving rumble deep in his chest. "Poor Miss Royalty. Is your whole life governed by the stuffy notions of long-faced eunuchs about what is proper?"

"Propriety is a becoming virtue in a woman, and absolutely imperative in a royal princess." She sounded like a prim mistress of protocol delivering a holy law.

Silver and black danced across his face like the rippling coat of some exotic running animal. Was he smiling at her?

"Princess, how old are you?"

"Twenty. I'll soon be twenty-one," she was quick to inform him.

"Twenty," he mused, yes, definitely smiling at her. "And I'll bet you've never even been kissed."

Dia's outrage halted her in the moon-spun shadows . . . and a sudden leaping fear.

"You . . . you're *drunk!*"

"Well, have you?"

"That is none of your concern." She walked on.

"Oh, well, I guess I'm right, if you won't answer."

"I don't answer because I'm not required to parade my personal life about for your inspection."

"You're afraid to answer."

"I am not."

"Yes, you are, because I'm right. You're twenty years old and never been kissed. Poor virtuous Miss Prim and Proper."

She whirled about to face him indignantly. "Oh, I have never met such an arrogant know-it-all! Well, I realize this will be difficult for you to believe, but you're *wrong!* I most certainly *have been kissed!*"

He feigned astonishment beneath his grin.

"Oh? Pecks on the cheek by doddering old senators and fancy court dandies?"

"A Captain of the Protectors!"

"Ha! A Protector! I knew it! Some dandied-up popinjay!"

"He was not—!

"And a captain, no less! Worse! Some perfumed aristocrat strutting about like a white-plumed peacock! Escorting the Imperial darling to and from her marble baths!" Atawulf, surprised at the jealous pang that vision caused him, retreated into sarcasm. "And did Your Royalty reward him with a kiss?"

Dia countered his sarcasm with frosty contempt. *"He* was a *gentleman!* His manners were impeccable and his virtue above reproach, which is more than you can claim."

"Oh, pardon me, Your Impeccable Royalty—"

"Stop calling me that."

"I'll bet he was a credit to his class." Atawulf snickered. "I'll bet he even wrote *love* poetry to you."

"What if he did?"

"Ah, he *did!* This is richer every moment. I'll bet you loved it—the honeyed praises of a lovesick pretty-boy."

"I knew it was a mistake to answer you at all."

He stood in the shadows, gazing down at her.

"Your mistake," he said softly, "was in lying to me."

"I haven't lied. What do you mean?"

"Aye, you did. If a lovesick Captain of the Protectors is all you've kissed—then you've never been kissed."

"Why, that's the most absurd, conceited—"

His hands rose to clasp her bare arms in palms strong and warm. His sudden touch sent shivers through her.

"Don't . . ."

"Dia." He spoke her name like a caress, husky and low. Slowly, deliberately, he bent toward her, his eyes holding her gaze.

She wanted to turn her face away, but she was drawn into those dark midnight eyes.

"Dia," he whispered.

She raised her face to his almost without realizing it, almost instinctively, the "oh" of astonishment still rounding her lips.

At first touch, his lips were warm, almost as soft as the moonlight, as velvety as the night, and she succumbed to the sensation.

As his kiss became more sure, as his mouth lingered over the sensitive fullness of her lips, the pleasant tingling sensation she felt became, without warning, hot and soaring. Her head tipped back and she was swept into a delicious slow spinning feeling that had nothing to do with the wine.

Atawulf, surprised by the unexpected warmth and melting of the ice princess, deepened his kiss, reveling in the sensation of touching her at last. How long had he been hungry for her? How long had he been denying his hunger?

As he delighted in the intoxicating feel and smell of her, his lips became more insistent. His hands slid around her slender waist, caressing the narrow of her back and pressing her closer. One hand moved up her spine to the smooth bare flesh just below the nape of her neck, twining his fingers in fallen strands of silky hair.

He pulled her toward him, encircled her, wanting every living inch of her.

And Dia felt as though she were melting into his embrace, this head-spinning kiss. She felt the strength in his hands pulling her close, the pressure of his hard-muscled body. And in his devouring desire she felt a pull, a need she had never experienced. Deep down she ached, and his warm, insistent, urging body was all that could assuage that ache.

This hot, newly awakened passion stunned her, frightened her, and with a gasp of panic she twisted her face aside, separating their lips. Her hands pushed against his massive chest, struggling to wrench free of his powerful arms.

Atawulf released her abruptly, and she fell away, staring up at him wide-eyed, shock and fear in her pale oval face. Reaching for her, he cursed inwardly when she backed away, staring at him as if he were the devil himself. And could he blame her? In a space of seconds passion had nearly overcome him. What in God's name did he expect? That she would throw herself upon him like some lusty wench? He had terrified her.

And Dia, breathing hard and peering up at his unreadable face in the shadow of the moon, wondered if she could ever face him by light of sun again after she so shamelessly responded to his kiss.

She raised the thin palla, which had slipped from her shoulders, and fled him, running through the trees like some lovely, elusive moon goddess whom he had violated and offended for all time.

And as he watched her disappear into her coach, followed by the darker form of Thalia, he heard a faint sliding sound and caught a glint of gold as something fell into the grass at his feet.

In his fingers was twined a glittering chain, a strand as fine as a spider's web. He bent to retrieve what had slid off the chain and found a tiny gold locket, almost a child's trinket. He closed his palm around the keepsake. It was still warm from lying next to her heart. And Bold Wolf never knew his arms could feel so empty as they did now.

• • •

Atawulf scratched at the oxhide flap of Alaric's tent. No light glimmered from within, but he was sure he had heard soft voices and rustlings. Now all was quiet.

"Alaric," he called again.

Silence seemed to hold its breath from within the tent, but Atawulf had been walking and thinking about this for half the night, and he would not be deterred.

Within the dark tent Winnifreya sat listening stark-still and perfectly naked atop her husband. Then she leaned over him, her long hair rippling over his bare chest, and tickled his earlobe with her tongue. Aroused, he shuddered beneath her, enjoying her temptings while trying to lie soundless and still.

"*Alaric!*" her brother's voice persisted from without.

Winnifreya murmured low and teasing to her husband. "If you get up, I'll bite your ear."

There, Atawulf knew he heard whispering from inside the tent.

"Alaric, I need to talk to you." His ears strained into the silence.

"*Ow!*" came a yelp of pain from within. "*Winn!*"

Shrieks of unsuppressed giggles burst from Atawulf's two nieces, and suddenly the Bold Wolf grinned, guessing what he had probably interrupted.

Alaric flung aside the tent flap, fingering his earlobe gingerly, and stepped outside. His nude body gleamed faintly with sweat and starlight, the cool air rapidly diminishing the proof that Atawulf's guess was correct.

"Atawulf, I assume this is important."

"It is."

"All right. Let's hear it."

Bold Wolf took a deep breath. "Find someone else to take charge of Princess Placidia. I want you to release me from that duty."

Alaric expelled a grunt of disbelief.

"You called me out in the middle of . . . of *sleep* to tell me that! This can wait until tomorrow." He turned and lifted the tent flap.

"No, it can't," said Atawulf, grasping his arm. "I have to know tonight—now—that she'll no longer be my responsibility."

At that Alaric snorted, but he turned back to his foster brother, alerted by the agitation in his voice.

"I know she's a pain in the ass and a tart-tongued little pest, but you don't seem to have any trouble with her. Why this aversion all the sudden? Why now?"

"Because . . . I can't be trusted with her."

Alaric stared at him briefly. "Atawulf, you're the *only* man who can be trusted with her."

"Not anymore. Not now."

With a huge sigh and a regretful glance toward the tent, Alaric clapped him on the shoulder. "Let's sit down." He nudged Atawulf in the direction of several black clumps in the dark.

"Over here." A plank of wood formed a bench between a tree stump and a barrel. Alaric sat down incautiously, and leapt up again as his bare bottom met splintered wood.

He swore expressively.

"Not your night, Alaric."

"It was, until you got a thorn under your saddle." He jerked down a horse blanket which was airing out over a tree limb and flung it over the bench. Now he sat safely, and Atawulf joined him.

"All right, brother. Why can't you be trusted with her?"

"Tonight I forced myself on her. Before I realized it I was kissing her."

"And . . . ?"

"And . . . she ran from me."

"That's it? You kissed her?"

"Aye, that's it, but . . . I didn't want to stop. It took all my will to let her go."

Alaric's teeth gleamed whitely in the dark as he grinned at his brother.

"You're a man, Atawulf, and for all her faults, Galla Placidia is a delicious eyeful of a woman." He chuckled. "And a handful, no doubt. But I believe Her Royal Snit has found her match in you."

Atawulf shook his head. "She's Roman, Alaric. And a royal hostage. It has to stay that simple."

"Are you in love with her?"

"God, no! How could I love a Roman? Tonight I just . . . I *wanted* her."

"Who do you suggest I put in charge of her? Sigeric?"

"*No!*"

"I'm jesting, brother. I know how Miss Priss would fare with Sigeric."

"Be serious. How about Wallia? He's half-smitten by her already. You saw his courtly show tonight."

"*You* be serious. She'd wrap poor Wallia around her dainty little finger and dangle him like a puppet."

Atawulf smiled at the notion. "Aye, she would, too."

"No, I'm afraid 'tis *you,* brother." Alaric slapped him on the shoulder and stood. His voice sobered. "The truth is you're the only man I really trust with this hostage. *If* anyone would bargain for her, they'd want her as virgin as the day we took her. And since her brother doesn't seem to want her back, she may be with us for a long time. But I'm gambling she'll be worth something to *someone* before this is over."

"Over," echoed Atawulf. "Will this ever be over, Alaric? Or will we wander homeless and landless till the end of our lives? How long before 'tis over?"

Alaric stood silent under the stars for a long moment. Finally he answered.

"If Rome won't come to a treaty, it won't be over until we destroy Rome or Rome destroys us."

Atawulf sighed heavily. "You know we won't destroy Rome, brother. So what does that leave?"

"You're tired, Atawulf."

"Aye, I'm tired. Tired of running and fighting and looting and moving on again. Tired of looking over my shoulder with no place to rest. We move and move, but the road just gets longer and rougher."

"Aye," Alaric nodded. "I spend sleepless nights wondering what to do next for all these people who depend on me. No answer is ever enough. I'm doing all I know to do, Atawulf. When we reach Rhegium with the rest of the hostages . . ." The King of the Goths shrugged.

"I know," Atawulf grimaced. "We'll move on."

7

At first light Atawulf pounded on the door of the royal coach to tell Dia to be ready—the Goths were moving on.

"Wait," she called through the door, then appeared tousled and sleepy-eyed. "Can't you hold up a bit?"

"Hold up? No, we can't."

"Please, you *must!*" she cried.

"Woman, what could be so important that you'd expect me to hold up forty thousand people?"

"I . . . I must go back to the garden. I lost something there."

"Is this what you lost?" Atawulf reached into a pouch slung to his belt and opened his hand. On his callused palm lay her golden locket.

"Why, yes!" she said, wide awake now.

He poured the chain and locket into her outstretched palm, careful that their hands did not touch.

Dia rubbed her thumb over the familiar surface, the artful etchings all but worn away with loving handling. She raised her eyes to him.

"It was a gift from my mother."

"I know."

"You opened it?"

"Aye, I confess I did." He had examined the keepsake and studied the portrait painted in gold on glass—a beautiful woman with gentle golden eyes.

"I knew you'd miss it," said Atawulf.

"Thank you," Dia said gratefully. "I could bear to lose anything but this. It's all I have of her." She opened the tiny clasp and gazed at the beloved face. "I've almost forgotten what she looked like, but for this picture. It reminds me."

"She's beautiful," said Atawulf.

"She was even more beautiful than this."

Atawulf looked up from the portrait to Dia, her soft curls honey gold in the breaking dawn and tousled around her lustrous eyes. *Aye, if she was half as beautiful as her daughter.*

Aloud he asked, "How old were you? When she died?"

"Four." She closed the locket carefully. The ineffable sadness in her face made him brusque.

"Aye, 'tis a great loss for a child." He recalled she had lost her father young, also. "I just came by to warn you we're moving. And to see if you suffered no . . . ill effects from last night. The wine, I mean."

"Oh! No! No ill effects." She felt very foolish and awkward, not knowing whether she flushed from embarrassment or some other turbulent emotion. She nearly stumbled over her words. "And you? No ill effects?"

"Me? Oh, no, not me."

She looked at him, waiting for she knew not what. Atawulf turned abruptly, as though he might walk away and say nothing more. But he came back, looking at her with lowered brows.

"Princess, I apologize for last night. I was forward and overbearing."

"You *were* forward," she teased with a lilt in her voice.

"I crossed all bounds of honor and . . . decency. I was drunk."

"Oh, well, I might have been . . . I mean, I didn't really . . ."

"It won't happen again. My oath on it."

"Oh."

She smoothed her skirt meticulously. "Of course. I suppose it shan't. How good of you to reassure me."

Atawulf looked relieved. "I just want you to understand. I didn't know what I was doing."

"I understand perfectly." Her voice was sharp with pique. "I believe you've sufficiently established that if you were in your right mind, you would certainly *never* have kissed me."

"You know, I'm trying to make a simple apology here, and you could accept it with a little more good grace. Good God, woman, I didn't commit murder! All I did was kiss you!"

"Which you seem to regret deeply. I've been kissed *before,* you know. No apology is necessary. *You're* the one making such a fuss over it."

He glared at her in exasperation and made as if to stalk away. In two strides he was back. "Well, don't worry, Miss Uppity. I won't make any more fuss!" He strode away again and almost immediately returned. "There won't be anything else to make a fuss about!"

She glared, her eyes fury-green. "I don't know why you're so angry. *You're* the one who crossed the bounds of decency. I think you owe me an apology!"

"Dammit, woman, I *did* apologize!" His blue eyes were disbelieving and wild.

"Then you ought to apologize for the way you apologized!" She stepped back into the coach and slammed the door.

Bold Wolf stared dumbfounded at the slammed door and

shuttered coach. Finally he turned away and flung his hands apart in hopeless appeal to the heavens.

"What did I say?"

The Gothic nation moved on with all speed southward, to what purpose Dia could not fathom. Perhaps Alaric's only interest was the winter stores of southern Italia, for he had an ever-growing number to feed, due to his impractical habit of taking in every liberated slave of Germanni blood who came to him.

As the weather cooled, the Gothic warriors denuded the country of grain and oil, sheep and cattle, and of course wine, leaving ravaged land behind them like locusts. They emptied the storehouses of the autumn harvest; they took their ease in villas and farm estates; they looted gold by the wagonload; they made use of the women as it pleased them. The unarmed people, protected from invasion for centuries by the legions, had no recourse but to let the Goths have their way.

Dia saw things outside her coach windows which sickened her. Dead men at the side of the road, men foolish enough or brave enough or angry enough to defy the barbarians. Country youths, girls and boys, frightened and trembling, rounded up and taken as slaves for the invaders. A burning village, from which the folk had fled with all the food they could carry in their escape, villages emptied and burned by the savage, relentless tide of devastation that was the Gothic army.

On this hasty march Dia saw Atawulf only at a distance; she had more time than she wished to dwell on that night in the garden. Thank God she had Thalia to talk to.

Just the two of them closeted in the royal coach, late at night, all around them the Gothic camp rustling and creaking in its restless way, at these times Dia confessed her innermost secrets.

"Oh, Thalia, it really *was* like I'd never been kissed. With Atawulf . . . he made me want to know what it feels like . . . you know, between a man and a woman." She lay on her back, staring up into the blackness toward the ceiling of the coach. "I think I almost would have let him . . . if he'd kissed me any longer . . . I wonder what would have happened."

"You know what would happen, Mistress Dia. He would've done what men do, and you'd have been plucked."

"Thalia! Who taught you to talk so vulgar?"

The slave girl cleared her throat hesitantly. "Dulcie, miss."

"I might have known. Well, believe me, I will not be *plucked* by a barbarian vagabond, no matter how handsome or manly. He . . . he caught me by surprise, that's all. I . . . I didn't know it would feel like . . . you know."

Thalia shook her head, unseen in the dark coach. No, she did not know. Careless flirtation had never entered her sheltered life as constant companion to the Imperial Princess. Few men dared or were in a position to approach her, and even fewer ever saw a flicker of interest in those solemn jet-dark eyes.

"Perhaps," Thalia whispered into the darkness, "perhaps he's in love with you."

"What! Oh, what utter nonsense, girl!" Dia laughed wildly, then fell silent. After a moment she said, "What makes you say that?"

"The way he looks at you, miss."

"That's his duty, looking after me. He's supposed to."

"With that hungry look in his eyes?"

"He's a man, isn't he? They all get that hungry look; it doesn't mean *love*."

Thalia hesitated, then said softly into the dark. "You let him kiss you an awfully long time before you broke away, miss."

"Oh, Thalia, I don't know what happened to me. I . . . I didn't want him to stop. But I simply *can't* fall in love with a Goth. I absolutely forbid myself to do any such thing. Besides, Atawulf doesn't love me. He was drunk; it never would have happened otherwise. You heard him say so. And I guess I was drunk, too."

She chuckled at the memory. "I've been cooped up in this coach too long. I'm no better than a randy peasant girl."

Queen Winnifreya and Singledia the Elder arrived unannounced before Placidia's coach one evening. Dia, surprised and pleased, sent Thalia to the door to invite them inside.

Winnifreya shook her fair head and Singledia's old voice rasped out like a scolding crow.

"Galla Placidia, this is no social call. Come out here, young woman. You've work to do."

More curious than intimidated, Dia emerged to stand on the lowered coach steps. She faced the two women, staring from one to the other, then she answered the eldest with a wry half-smile. "Have you decided I've not enough to do to keep me out of idleness? Have you brought me your laundry, perhaps?"

Singledia the Elder's keen old eyes narrowed and she spoke sharply and to the point. "You've neglected your duties long enough, Princess of the Romans. I thought you'd come to them on your own—they're your people, you'd have to care about how they fare."

"Pardon me, but I'm sure I don't know what, or whom, you're referring to."

"I don't doubt that, but 'tis something you'll remedy if you ever expect to make an Empress."

Dia did not bother to correct the old woman's misconception; she was curious to learn what Atawulf's mother thought an Empress ought to be doing that Dia was not.

"All right. Tell me how I may redeem myself in your opinion, Lady Singledia."

"Not by calling me high-flung titles, you won't. Those don't carry water with me. Only by your acts, like the Gospel says, will you show if you be good fruit or bad."

"What is it I've done?"

"You've done nothing—that's the trouble. There's Roman folk out there you pretend to care so much about, and you've not so much as asked to see them and find out how they are and give them any reason to think their own royal princess has a care for their welfare."

"Why, you mean the hostages? I spoke to Alaric about them and he assured me—"

"But did you bother to assure them?"

"Why, no, I . . . I didn't think it was necessary. Aren't they taken care of?"

"You don't even know, do you? You're the one person they ought to be able to depend on to see to them."

"It has never been my duty to *see* to people, Singledia."

"Then just what do you think *is* your duty to your people?"

Dia stood silent. She did not really know what sort of duty she had that would be worth much to this crusty old Goth. Being an example of virtue and propriety seemed rather silly. As a mere princess, she didn't make laws or decrees or taxes. In fact, she always had an idea that the people had a duty to her—to show her deference, to come out to see her when she passed in her carriage, to bow and show her respect.

Dia had an uneasy feeling that Singledia would demand to know *why* they owed her respect, and she knew the fact that she was daughter and granddaughter to emperors would not be enough for the mother of Atawulf and Winnifreya.

She took a deep breath. "The truth is, someone else has always seen to the people."

"Who?"

"I don't know . . . the magistrates, the governors, the prefects."

Singledia looked around. "No magistrates or prefects here."

Dia stepped down from the steps onto the dusty ground. "Perhaps," she said quietly, "you will take me to them."

"Oh, aye, I intend to."

Dia threw her palla over her head, for autumn was brisk in the air. Her hair was unbound, the amber-brown tresses whisking from beneath the palla to dance in the wind.

She accompanied the royal Gothic women through the camp, which was a chaotic sprawl of exhausted and hungry folk hastily unhitching wagons and starting cookfires. Many people scarcely noticed them, but some waved or called a greeting to the women. And Dia noticed that Winnifreya, as well as her mother, always smiled and returned the greeting, often even stopping to speak with various folk along the way.

Winnifreya glanced sideways toward the Imperial Princess. "We are taking you to speak to your people, Placidia. I'm surprised you've not asked to see them before now. Surely I'm mistaken in thinking you do not care to speak to the women and children we hold hostage."

"It is not the custom of the Imperial family to go among the people as though they were our equals, as you do. They come to see us in royal processions; we are not required to condescend to them."

"Condescend? Are you implying that speaking to my people is condescending to them? I live among them and care about them. These are my people, my brothers and sisters and cousins."

Winnifreya halted on the dead dry weeds they trod and turned to confront the shorter Roman. "These women are frightened and certain we mean harm to them and their children. All our assurances can never equal one word from you, Princess Placidia, if you will approach them with confidence, let them see that you have come to no harm at our hands, and assure them that they also will not. Will you do that for your people?"

"That depends, Queen of the Goths," Dia said levelly. "I will not lie to them, therefore I ask you—*will* they come to no harm? What is to become of them?"

Winnifreya nodded solemnly. "They are held for ransom—a ransom I cannot disclose to you or anyone as yet—but I can promise you they will be released safely when we reach our destination. Alaric will not murder them; he gives his word on that."

"And your word, Winnifreya?"

"And mine."

Now Dia nodded. "I will speak to them."

As they continued through the camp, Dia noted a look of approval on Singledia's wrinkled face, and she felt taller, walked more surely. Why the approval of an old barbarian woman should make the daughter of emperors glow with pride was a question she dismissed as quickly as it crossed her mind. It mattered. No court training had ever prepared her for this . . . this being flung out on her own, no courtiers, officials, or clerks to hasten to her bidding, to strew their bureaucratic ramparts, ditches, and stakes between her cozy palace and the rest of the world.

There were only the Goths and frightened Roman captives and herself, alone, with no protocol to guide her—or inadequate protocol, for she suspected she would be forbidden to concern herself *personally* with merchants' wives and lesser nobility.

But Singledia, mother of two warriors and a queen, foster mother to a king, expected Placidia to live up to her royal blood, to prove she deserved the legacy of Valentinian and Theodosius, of Justina and Galla. Strength, courage, and pride, Singledia had demanded, but there was something more that Placidia knew she had left unspoken. What was it? Duty? Responsibility? Neither of those words sounded strong enough or deep enough.

The captives were corralled near the center of the Gothic camp. The wagons needed to carry two hundred women and children were roped off from the rest of the camp, guarded by a score of warriors. Within the circle the captive women struggled to stew grain and vegetables in a great copper cookpot over a campfire. Children gathered deadwood and carried baskets of stale bread passed to them over the slender rope barrier.

As the captives caught sight of the delegation of women approaching them, they straightened and stared, and Dia saw that they wore dresses and cloaks which once had been fine and costly but now hung limp, bedraggled, and torn. Their noble-born children looked like beggar brats, dirty and unkempt; they scuffled up to the edge of the circle to stare at the visitors.

Now she was close enough to see the women's faces clearly, their expressions as individual as the spirits behind them: faces pale and frightened; faces sullen, defiant, proud; faces weary, empty of hope; faces calm, determined, strong.

Dia halted just outside the rope, and the women slowly moved toward her. There was no reason for them to know who she was. Likenesses of the emperor's half-sister did not exist outside of a few tiny portraits painted for family members.

No, the Roman women should not have known her, yet they did. First one bowed, then another, until all of them, unpracticed and fumbling, had lowered their heads before her.

Then they stood and watched her, women and children, silent and solemn, eyes somber and fearful. They looked to her as if she had some hope for them, some answer to the questions in those anxious eyes. And the something more she felt was not duty or responsibility, but something indeed deeper and stronger. If she had stopped to put a name to it she would have called it *compassion*.

Dia's heart went out to them. In a sudden breach of protocol, she ducked under the rope and approached them, palms open in greeting. She had never addressed the people directly, never consorted with commoners, but these were captives, hostages like herself, and she knew their fears, their uncertainties, their losses.

Roman women, her own people, looking to her with hope and fear, trust and desperation.

"Sisters," she said quietly, remembering the simple greeting used in the devout House of Marcella. "I've been remiss in not coming before now. How do you fare? Are you well treated?"

Suddenly they were all around her, some even touching her, the words tumbling from them all together in a jumble of noise. "Our men are released—why did they not let us go, too? Why are they keeping us? What will happen to us? Where do they take us? What will they do to the children?"

Dia hastened to reassure them. Alaric had given his word, she said, that they would not be harmed, and Winnifreya had given her word as well.

"I believe you are in no danger, nor your children. I have the promise of the King and Queen of the Goths, whose word I trust in full faith."

She did not see the soft glow in the queen's eyes in response to her words, nor the approving smile of the older woman. Her attention was full on the hostages, who now plied her with plaintive woes.

"I am ill, nobilissima, and they sent me a horse doctor! We've had no baths, nor a change of clothes, and we've been here a week! My children have only sandals, and the weather is turning cold! Look what they give us to eat!"

"I will find you a physician," she told them, "and see to shoes for your children." But then she chuckled gently. "As for the food, I'm likely having the same supper as you are. It isn't fancy, I'll grant you, but it's filling—and healthier than some of the banquets I've tasted."

Then they warmed her heart with the questions which followed. "Are you well, nobilissima? Do they treat you as they ought? Is it true they refuse to return you to the Emperor? Will you be released with us?"

"No," she answered gravely, "I do not believe I am to be released with you." Then she gave a little rueful smile. "Actually I believe the Goths would very much like to return me to the Emperor, but it seems my brother thinks they ask too high a ransom."

The women expressed shock and sympathy. Dia, unaccustomed to being the recipient of sympathy, and feeling slightly embarrassed, glanced outside the rope circle toward Singledia and Winnifreya. Suddenly her heart beat out of time.

There sat Atawulf upon his great red war-horse, leaning forward with one arm propped upon his thigh, watching her with his keen blue gaze, eyes intent beneath his craggy brows.

Her pulse quickened at the sight of him, then the fact that she reacted so ridiculously irked her. Flustered, she turned her back on him, turned her flushed face to the Roman women, hoping that he had not noticed the effect he had on her, fervently hoping no one had noticed.

She made her farewell to the captives, promising to see to their needs and to return on the morrow, but her mind strayed to the thought of Atawulf behind her, those blue eyes burning into her, and she scarcely knew what she said. But when she turned to duck under the rope again, he was gone.

In the days and weeks which followed she saw little of Atawulf, for the Goths were on the move. When he rode up on Red Demon to see that nothing was amiss, he never dismounted but remained unerringly polite. She, too, could be cool and correct, like any court-bred young woman, but she looked forward with restless anticipation to his morning visits.

If she caught an unexpected glimpse of him out riding with his small son, or cantering off somewhere beside Alaric or Wallia, she would catch her breath and almost forget to breathe again until he had ridden out of sight. She would shake her head and laugh at her childish reaction to his mere presence. His mere existence. For she thought of him more often than she ought, more often than he warranted. It was a good thing, she told herself, that he was so distracted and distant, giving her no chance to make a fool of herself . . . a fool over a man who had simply once gotten drunk and kissed her.

I will not fly into a passion over a barbarian, over a Goth, over some half-dressed savage called Bold Wolf.

Bold Wolf had his hands full day and night, with one crisis after another in the Gothic caravan, which was just as well with him. It gave him less time to dwell on *her*. Since seeing her among the women hostages, hearing her reassure them and speak to them as though the chasm of rank between them did not exist, he had felt his heart wrenching open to her again, despite his determination to chain it fast.

Then she had caught him gazing at her and immediately turned her back on him. Abruptly and starkly he was reminded that she was not for him, that the chasm between them was less easily crossed than the chasm of rank. They were Goth and Roman, their races adamantly and irreversibly opposed.

Yet he could not bring himself to send a captain or a lieutenant to check on her in his stead. He tortured himself with that daily morning visit, but he kept his distance, riding Demon beside the bouncing, creaking coach, senselessly fueling the flame of his fever with the sight of her face framed in the swaying window, her voice low and careful as she answered his queries.

He rode apart, keeping away from her, so that if he should unknowingly carry the sickness the Goths suffered, he would not pass it to her. It had been a scorching summer followed by a dry autumn, the days crisp and crackling, parched. The rivers they found were shrunken, sluggish and warm, sometimes brackish green and scummy around the sides. Sickness, a burning fever and thirst with a cramping vise in the guts, vomiting and voiding, took hold of many of the wanderers.

Then, at last, in November, it rained.

The clouds blew up, piling and muttering and glowering, until they burst loose with torrents of blinding, stinging rain, cold and unrelenting. The cracked-earth lowlands the caravan crossed suddenly became a chill marshland, a cold, treacherous bog. They traveled in a long, wet line, battling to keep horses, cattle, and sheep on the highway and out of the sucking mud and sudden wild-raging floods.

And all this time Alaric, sick with the fever himself, pushed Atawulf, pushed them all to reach their destination before winter, for it was imperative to Alaric's plan that they not delay.

While Alaric, pale and unsteady in the saddle, strove to ride about camp and give encouragement to the sick and the well alike, Bold Wolf tried to be everywhere at once, tried to solve every problem, handle every crisis, carry every burden himself, before word of any of it came to his foster brother. Atawulf and Wallia were determined to take every task from Alaric's shoulders and mind, and Winnifreya did the same for her part, while struggling with the still harder task of persuading her husband to rest.

He did not rest, but came down with chills and a sweating fever, which put him flat on his back in a wagon. To keep him abed, Atawulf pressed the Goths onward, pushing and pulling, goading and cajoling and encouraging, though he was weary to the bone himself. The Goths made slow progress down the coast, with so many of them ill, and the rain, once started, never seemed to let up long enough for them to dry out. The heavy blanket of clouds overhead so obscured the sun that, for all they knew, it had been drowned to a cold cinder.

They were fortunate, Atawulf thought with gloomy irony, covering his head with the hood of a woolen cloak heavy with rainwater, that the Emperor was a fool and a coward and no legions pursued them, for the Goths would have been hard put to battle fresh soldiers fed by steady supply lines.

And as if he did not have enough on his mind, his thoughts continually strayed to the royal occupant of the Imperial coach. He cursed himself for a fool whenever he caught himself reliving that night, remembering the feel and the smell and the look of her in the moonlight, the sudden yielding of her lips, the press of her warm body against his, the curve of her round hips beneath his hand, the smooth silkiness of her skin.

He shook the memory off like shaking water off a sodden cloak. She was angry with him for that kiss, and he could not blame her—she practically had to fight him off before he came to his senses. If she seemed cool and distant now, impeccably polite, it was no more than he deserved. He was angry with himself, too—

angry with himself for forgetting that she was a Roman and an Imperial Princess of that arrogant breed, spoiled and haughty and not about to suffer the touch of a dirty barbarian brigand.

He was too old for brooding over a woman—especially this woman, whom he reminded himself he didn't want and who wanted none of him, either. The best thing that could happen, he thought as he trudged through the muddy camp, would be for Alaric to trade her off to her brother and be done with her. Then he could shrug her out of his memory forever.

Dia lay in the night listening to the endless rain splattering, splattering atop the coach. She wrapped her comforter closer about her in the November chill, eyes open in the dark, wide awake—driven by idle days and restless nights to tossing from thought to tumbling thought.

Would the rain ever stop? Would they ever reach a destination? Could she bear being cramped in this coach another day? Another night?

Her body lay perfectly still, but her mind spun in interminable circles.

She wondered, what was *he* doing at this time of night? What did he think about? Did he ever think about that evening in the garden? Surely he did; his kiss had been too urgent, too sensuous to forget. Unless it had been what he said—a drunken whim.

As she remembered his touch, her mouth tasting his, a river of warmth spread through her body. His hands on her had been strong and roughened with hard work; his kiss, at first tender and exploring, had suddenly become devouring.

When she recalled the feel of his iron-muscled arms holding her against the hard flesh of his thigh, she blushed in the dark, heat coursing from somewhere deep inside her, sending hot waves through her whole body, and she shuddered again, turned to her side and curled up in a little ball, for that feeling would pulse and grow within her and she did not want it to. That feeling made her long for something she should not want—something she refused to want: his touch, his hands and mouth and body on hers.

I will not be brought low by an unruly body, she told herself in the dark. *We are worlds apart, enemies, and he wants me no more than I want him.*

The best thing that could happen to her, she told herself grimly, was for the Goths to trade her back to her brother and send her home to her own people, her own world—the sooner the better.

Dia stared amazed at the multitude of ships, a flotilla of merchant, grain, and fishing vessels dipping and rising in the sparkling harbor, the water of the strait a flawless blue under a clear, cool winter sky.

"Just look at all the ships!" Dia breathed. "Have you ever seen so many? Such a magnificent picture. And look there—the water is ripples of sapphire and crystal!"

Craft of all sizes and shapes crowded the harbor at Rhegium: long, sleek sailing ships with triangular topsails; wide-beamed single-masted fishing boats; round-hulled deep-bottomed cargo ships; vessels with single and double masts, large and small square sails, most of the canvas furled but a few displaying their colorful stripes and emblems.

Dia's only companions on the breezy terrace overlooking the harbor were Thalia, Priscus Attalus, the ever-present Captain Rayard, and a handful of guards.

Priscus Attalus was not so taken with the sight. "Strange, don't you think, nobilissima? Winter is the most dangerous season for sailing, yet here is gathered a veritable fleet."

Placidia looked at the old ex-Senator, ex-pretender to the purple, considering the import of his words. Then she turned back to the incredible array of ships on the water.

"Alaric," she said, certainty strong in her voice.

"I fear so."

"This is his ransom for the women and children."

"He is releasing them today," confirmed Attalus.

She raised her eyes, her gaze sweeping past the rocky coast surrounding the harbor. The winter air was so pristine, it seemed to sharpen the far view; across the shimmering blue strait the craggy headlands of Sicilia stood crisp and clear against a cloudless sky. The distant shore seemed so close she imagined she could smell the pines upon the high slopes.

Sicilia, across the narrow strait, would be Alaric's destination. He had brought his wandering Goths to Rhegium, the very boot-tip of Italia, to float them across to the mountainous island. This time of year the grain houses would be bursting with the wheat harvest, the fruits and wine would be stored.

Aloud she said, "So Alaric thinks to pillage Sicilia. Is this the great plan he's been so secretive about? The stores may last the Goths the winter, but then what? And while he sits on that island, what's to prevent my brother sending the navy to trap him?"

Priscus Attalus's bald dome gleamed in the sunlight as he shook his head. He answered her heavily.

"I'm afraid Sicilia is not his final destination, nobilissima."

"Naturally. He'll have to return come spring."

"No, he'll take the harbors and shipyards. Alaric has once before tried forcing me to persuade the Senate to turn a fleet of galleys over to him."

"Galleys? For what purpose?"

"He claimed he meant to free Rome from the grain blockade. He planned to sail to Africa and capture the storehouses, then bring home the wheat to Rome. He purported to save the city from starvation."

"Oh, what twisted logic! He had only to lift the siege and take his beggar army elsewhere, and my brother would have allowed the grain shipment."

"As I told the Senate," Attalus acknowledged. "On my advice, they refused Alaric the ships."

Dia laughed huskily. "So that's why Alaric demoted you, old fox. You were a puppet whose strings he couldn't pull."

The old statesman drew himself up proudly, grasping his cloak at the breast as though he wore a toga. "I have never in my life been anyone's puppet, Most Noble Placidia. Nor am I such a traitor to the Empire that I would allow barbarians to seize control over her grainlands."

"Yes," said Dia thoughtfully. "My father knew well that he who controls the grain controls the Empire. It is not idle whim that to give a ship to a barbarian is a crime punished by death. You think Alaric still hopes to carry out his scheme—to take Africa?"

"Aye," spoke a sudden voice behind them. "You may be sure of it."

They spun to face Atawulf, who had come silent as a stalking leopard onto the terrace.

"And Egypt as well," grinned Atawulf, "if I know Alaric."

Dia stared at him stonily. "You'll never reach Africa with this motley collection of boats. You'll be trapped on Sicilia."

Atawulf jutted his beard at her, baiting her. "We'll have the shipyards, and the shipbuilders will build whatever we need, there's no doubting that."

Dia was not to be baited. "This is the dream of desperation, Atawulf; you must know that. Even if you reach Africa, there are legions there who will stop you. Admit it; the Goths are still running. Once you cross these straits, you'll have no place left to retreat."

Those blue eyes darkened, a deep well of doubt, but in an instant anger glittered between the narrowed lids. Or was it defiance? She realized she had struck a vein of truth that Atawulf did not want mined.

"Where will the Goths go after this, Bold Wolf?" she asked more gently than she intended.

"Where do you suggest we stop?" he snapped. "Here? On these rocks, with naught but the sea before us and cold bogs behind? When you have an answer to that, woman, I will hear your opinion. Not before!"

She sucked in her breath, but she made no reply. There was no answer. She knew it, as did Atawulf. The Goths moved on because they had no choice. Alaric had led them into the heart of Italia, and now they had no retreat, no safe haven, except the hope of the Sicilian island and a vague dream of African grainlands.

Dia pressed her lips together and turned her gaze back out across the strait toward the distant line of cliffs. She tried to harden her heart. The Goths had gotten themselves into this hopeless position when they invaded Italia and laid siege to Rome. They deserved no sympathy from her. Why did she persist in feeling their pain—*his* pain?

Atawulf's gaze lingered along the delicate lines of her face profiled against sea and shoreline, and the sight of her called to him like a song from a forgotten homeland, opening his heart to that ache which he did not know how to ease.

He retreated within himself and pulled his gaze away from her, turning his eyes toward the sea, the craggy headlands, their destination.

"You're coming down to the shore," he told her roughly. "There's a house there where Rayard and his men will keep you closely guarded tonight. We sail with first light."

With a sharp nod to Rayard, Atawulf left the terrace. Dia did not turn until she was sure he was gone, then she took her leave of Attalus and accompanied Captain Rayard to her night's prison.

The house was not altogether a prison. It was a wealthy merchant's home near the harbor, confiscated for this night. The outer garden sloped down to a seaside chapel used by the fisherfolk, and Dia, restless, told Rayard that she wished to walk down to the chapel and pray.

Three of them walked through the silent garden—Placidia,

Thalia, and Captain Rayard—beneath a sky so clear and star-strewn it seemed they might reach out and gather sparkling handfuls.

The open doors of the chapel looked out to the sea, and within, light danced invitingly, like a beacon in the night, the glow of many candles—each warm flame set there by a reverent soul—illuminating the interior with a welcoming golden glow which paled the cold stars.

So the chapel seemed to Dia, in her need of comfort and counsel for her heart, and she gladly entered the light. She covered her hair with her woolen mantle and took an unlit candle from a box near the door.

Thalia hesitated in the doorway. "Mistress," she said, glancing over her shoulder to see if Rayard could hear, "I can't go in; I'm in my blood-flow."

"Oh." Dia had forgotten. "Thalia, no one's here, and besides, it isn't Mass."

"You know a woman shouldn't go unclean before God, Miss Dia. Suppose he won't hear your prayers if I'm with you."

Dia looked disappointed. "You'll have to wait outside then."

"Yes," Thalia said, trying not to sound too relieved. She hated prayer vigils. The Greek slave remembered far too many times when she had accompanied the princess during long vigils forced upon them by Serena, who believed hours of repentance was the quickest cure for frivolity in young girls.

Dia hated prayer vigils, too, but tonight she was confused and uncertain in her heart. Tonight her heart warred with her head, her feelings with her loyalties. She lit her small candle from a large one beside the altar. Candles glittered at the feet of the statues, making the painted features seem alive in their light: statues of Christ, of the Virgin, and of Saint John the Evangelist, the special protector of the fishermen and seafarers who used this harbor. By far the most candles lit the serene face of John the Beloved, the Son of the Thunderstorm—storms in the Strait of Messana being sudden and deadly in their fury—and Dia paused before him and silently asked of him safe passage tomorrow, protection upon the sea, though the voyage would be brief and the waters were calm tonight.

But her own candle she placed before the Virgin. She needed to speak with the Holy Mother, for Mary had been the recipient of many of her prayers and knew much of her heart and her dilemma. Dia sank to her knees on the stone floor and looked up into the gentle face of the Blessed Virgin.

Thalia strolled along the shore, breathing in the fresh salt air, turning her face toward the black sky, the starry infinity. She loved the open space above her, and before her the sound of surf surging, surging, upon a black line of breakers etched on the dark shifting sea.

The granddaughter of a Greek scholar-slave, Thalia loved the enormity of the universe. Out here in the night her soul seemed to expand to fill the vast spaces of existence.

The rocky path beneath her feet divided near an outcropping of boulders. The left-hand path continued along the beach, winding below the crags. The right-hand path climbed behind the rocks, leading up into dark brush and the shadows of trees.

Though she had told Captain Rayard that she was only going to walk along the beach a short while, Thalia picked up her skirts and set her sandals with care upon the upward path. Peering up the dark bluff, she thought she saw light flickering amid the trees, and was it her fanciful imagination that heard a faint rattle of drum and timbrel, a thin melody of flute, and faraway snatches of chanting? Or was it all part of the endless surging and murmuring of the waves?

She climbed easily in the dark, for the path was well-trodden, though she was nearly breathless when she reached the top of the rise. By now she knew the chanting and music were not her imagination, and she did not need the light of the rising crescent moon to make out the clearing in the scrub oaks, for it was lit by a fire within a small ring of rocks.

Before the fire stood a statue, the flickering orange light dancing upon the stone features of Rhea, the Great Mother, seated in a chariot. Two stone lions sat before her as if awaiting her word to leap the chariot out over the bluffs. The Goddess's high crown was shaped like the towers of cities, and in her hand she held a flat drum—a drum just like the one playing in the clearing now.

A score of women danced in a circle, naked women of all ages—lithe young girls stepped lightly beside wrinkled, sag-breasted grandmothers; maidens full-bosomed and round-bottomed linked hands with women thin from toil or ripe with child—all of them naked under stars and crescent moon and firelight. A trio of women played drum, timbrel, and flute, while the rest danced for the Mother Goddess.

Suddenly Thalia remembered: tonight was the winter solstice, and she had stumbled upon a rite as old as the sun and moon. This secret dance before Rhea was unlawful under Roman decree and unholy by Church edict, and Thalia knew she was witnessing a dying drama, a secret worship that whispered to her of her ancestors, of centuries past, reverence for the old gods of earth and air, fire and water, a dance of love for the mother of humankind, of life.

And it seemed appropriate to Thalia that this solstice rite took place on a high bluff overlooking the sea, on the edge of the cliffs above this wild strait of epic lore, as though the worship of the Goddess had been pushed to the edge of the world, and this isolated remnant of the old religion clung to this wild shore with no place left to retreat.

Slowly Thalia became aware of the words rising and falling on the wind, the chant of the women growing in strength and power.

Mother Sea . . . Mother Wave . . . Mother Sky . . .
Mother Wind . . . Mother Cloud . . . Mother Storm . . .
Sea Wave Sky . . . Wind Cloud Storm . . .
Drive the slayers from our shores . . .

Over and over, louder and louder, as the roundelay and the music grew wilder and wilder.

Mother Sea . . . Mother Wave . . . Mother Sky . . .
Mother Wind . . . Mother Cloud . . . Mother Storm . . .
Sea Wave Sky . . . Wind Cloud Storm . . .
Drive the slayers from our shores . . .

Suddenly one of the dancer's eyes were on her. An old woman, with eyes as silver as a cat's in torchlight. And as the naked crone's feet beat in rhythm as lively as a girl's, as she spun with linked hands about the circle, her eyes turned toward Thalia. Those old eyes, bright, vital, and keen, met hers full of challenge, full of mystery, full of *invitation*.

Thalia never knew why she turned and fled. Fear caught in her throat, though it was not fear of these pagan women, nor fear of a stone image. Perhaps a fear of what they represented—a wildness, an abandon to nature, a reveling in their very aliveness, their very creaturehood. And perhaps because they were a lost cause, a breed doomed to die a slow death, parched of the spirit, for the waters of the Empire would no longer nourish their kind, but rather poison them from bitter wells of ostracism and persecution.

Thalia fled down the dark path, stumbling in her haste and catching her flying hair in a low-hanging tree limb. This panicked her more than it should, for perhaps the dancers would chase after her, to silence her for having discovered their unlawful ritual. With a small cry she tore her hair free and staggered down the rocky trail.

A huge black figure loomed suddenly before her, and before she could halt her headlong flight arms reached out and caught her. Wildly Thalia struggled until the strong arms held her still and the voice penetrated her brain.

"Thalia! Thalia, stop! Who's after you? Are you all right?"

She sighed in relief and relaxed in Rayard's grip.

"What happened? Is someone chasing you?"

Thalia shook her head. Faintly above the surf she thought she could hear the drum beating in unbroken rhythm, but she could hear no chanting now.

"No one is chasing me."

"Then what are you afraid of?"

She gave a shaky little laugh. "I believe I frightened myself. I . . . my imagination has run wild."

"What were you doing up there? You said you'd only walk a ways along the beach. I was afraid something had happened to you."

She stared up at him, unable to make out his expression in the gloom. "You left Mistress Dia? You left her alone in the chapel?"

"Aye, looking for you. Come on, let's get back."

Rayard turned her down the trail, keeping his arm around her on the uneven path. The beach was but a short distance, and soon they were hurrying along the pebbled shore.

"Step lively, girl, before we're missed!" Rayard caught her hand and pulled her along at a fast pace.

"You shouldn't have come," Thalia panted beside him. "You shouldn't have left her."

"Aye, I'll catch hell from Atawulf if anything befalls her. And I'd catch hell from *her* if you fell off a cliff and broke your pretty neck. Oh, Lord, there's Atawulf. I'm in for it now!"

Where the hell is Rayard? Atawulf paced silently before the chapel. He stopped, half-hidden outside the doorway, and looked within. She was still there, her dark green cloak soft as moss in the candlelight. Her head bowed, she remained on her knees, praying.

He wondered what she prayed for. Probably that he and all the rest of the Goths would be swallowed up by the sea.

For the tenth time that night Atawulf inspected the sky. If the weather held they would have easy sailing. The stars still glittered as sharp and clear as the myriad candles in the chapel. Then he noticed a slight change in the south. The stars were dimmer than before, hazy, as if a thin cloud or fog drifted in off the sea.

Atawulf sniffed the air, and maybe he detected a heavy, moist smell, a change in the atmosphere. *'Twill be fog in the morning. Not too much, I hope.*

A scuffling sound on the beach startled him, and he spun about, prepared to draw his sword. Here came Rayard and Thalia—at a run.

Dia finally gave up and admitted that her pleas to the Blessed Mother were only half-hearted. She wanted to beg Mary's help in cleansing her soul and her thoughts.

She knew she should be praying for divine intervention, for the hand of God to halt the course of the barbarians.

But her thoughts kept straying to Atawulf. To the way his grin could light up her heart, when he wasn't being sarcastic. The way his blue eyes drew her into their rich depths and sometimes made her forget what she had been saying. The way sunlight danced off his hair and turned it to gold.

The way his laughter played upon her heart and his silence echoed hollow and lonely in her soul.

"Oh, Blessed Mary, I know I'm foolish, but I love him. Perhaps, just possibly, you could see him as I do and understand.

"My prayer may be unworthy and frivolous in your eyes, Holy Mother, but please, I think he might love me a little, too. If you could just open his heart a little, if you could just whisper in his ear . . .

"I'm but flesh and blood, Blessed Mother, as you were. You loved a man once, so I'm sure you cannot find offense in me for feeling as I do.

"And please, don't think me a traitor. I know the Goths should be stopped, but I cannot really hate them or wish them harm. They are good people, many of them. I believe they are simply desperate. If you could just somehow persuade my brother to come to fair terms with them, to give them a place to settle, then I believe they would change . . ."

She turned her head, diverted by raised voices outside the chapel. She thought she heard Atawulf growling and Rayard's croak of protest. Then she clearly heard Thalia enter the argument.

"Pardon me, Holy Mother," she said hastily, rising to her feet, "but I must go resolve whatever nonsense is going on outside. Amen."

Mist hovered over the strait, wrapping the opposite shore in a grey veil. The sun rose pale and white, an indistinct pearl, slowly lightening the sky. The air, motionless and wet, muted the slow beat of waves upon the rocks, muted even the stamping, thudding, shouting melee upon the docks.

Shivering, Dia pulled her cloak close against the morning chill. The sea looked peaceful this solstice, and the fog was lifting. The higher the sun climbed the sky, the more distinct became the dark line of cliffs directly across the water.

She could see Atawulf, his mane of hair pulled up and bound with red leather at the crown of his head so that it whipped like a proud horse's tail as he dashed here and there upon the piers, forging chaos into order, while hundreds of nervous horses and equally nervous men milled about.

Virtually none of the Goths had ever been aboard a ship, ever been on the sea, and these bobbing, swaying wooden vessels looked unsteady and unreliable to the horse warriors. But they steeled their nerves and led their blindfolded war-horses up the puny planks and onto the boats, while the hired sailors of the various craft glanced at each other knowingly and tried not to smirk at the barbarians.

The first wave of ships to set forth, the largest and sturdiest, would transport half the horses and riders and foot soldiers. They expected at least token resistance when they landed at Messana on the Sicilian shore, but they were prepared to battle a full garrison if necessary.

The women and children and old men prepared to embark on the second wave of vessels, followed by the rest of the warriors and horses. A few of these craft looked doubtful even to Dia. She glanced at Winnifreya and Singledia the Elder, who waited upon the terrace with her. The Queen of the Goths looked grim; her knuckles were mottled scarlet and white from gripping the balustrade.

At last, half the morning gone, the various cargo and fishing vessels began casting off, flashing oars and hoisting sails. Atawulf and Alaric each rode in a lead ship, planning to be the first to disembark and command their men in seizing the city.

By threes and fours the ships set off across the green sea under a pale sky mottled with grey clouds. The headlands directly across the water were clear now, grey and green, but the ships set their rudders northwest through the strait; it was seven miles sailing from Rhegium to Messana, seven miles from safe harbor to safe harbor, between the rugged crags and jagged breakers of the Strait of Messana.

The ships spread out on the water, colorful sails unfurled to catch what little southern breeze they might find, but the oarsmen propelled the vessels steadily toward the middle of the strait. Here the water was deep and wide and less swift than the dangerous narrows farther north.

Dia looked northward and saw a black line upon the horizon. She glanced at Thalia, but her handmaiden's attention was elsewhere. Thalia stared up the rocky cliff at the edge of the harbor, but when Dia followed her gaze she saw naught but a small congregation of peasant women huddled together on a bluff, clutching their homespun shawls and watching the ships set out.

No, not watching the ships, but looking north, beyond the growing flotilla spreading out across the strait. Dia's eyes followed the turn of their heads, and it seemed the black line above the headlands had grown in those few seconds, had expanded and ascended, skimming between the feathery grey clouds and the darkling sea.

The tide of cloud rolling toward them was an impenetrable black, blotting out the sky, eating up the day, bearing down upon them with alarmingly swift motion.

Dia thought she could hear the wind screaming. The black cloud, even as it came, churned in upon itself like a great wave, and though she saw no lightning, Dia heard a deep, distant rumble, and soon half the sky would be a black, raging storm.

Dia wasn't aware of her cry of dismay, until she saw both Winnifreya and Singledia staring at her with terror, their blue eyes almost colorless. Her hand flew to her mouth, her own eyes wide with horror. She turned from them and sought out the lead ships, far into the strait.

Already ships were turning about and struggling to return to Rhegium, and a fortunate few were close enough to the harbor, but for the rest it was too late, too late, as the cold winds and wild waves of the black storm sped upon them, a howling fury.

8

ATAWULF RAISED his eyes to the northern sky, and the black tide racing upon the wind froze his heart. Massive blue-black stormclouds roiled and churned toward them, obscuring the placid sky like smoke in a burning dome.

"Turn! Turn! Look what is upon us!"

His was not the only voice raised in panic. Already other cries joined his.

"About! About and give her your stern!"

"Trim sails!"

"Merciful Jesus!"

Atawulf looked to the man at the helm, who leaned on the tiller, holding it tucked beneath his arm, glancing up at the sky and grimly taking a firmer grip. Slowly, far too slowly, the ship struggled to turn from the nightmare rolling upon their heads.

Atawulf heard the scream of the wind before he felt the first cold breath lift his damp hair. Then a violent jolt shook the deck beneath his feet as the full force of the gale struck the sails, and the sea rocked the ship from bow to stern.

Water washed the deck. Braced for it, Atawulf held to the aft mast, while abruptly, above him, the violent headwind knocked their gentle tailwind out of the sails. For a fractured second the sails collapsed, then the canvas snapped, sharp, like a whipcrack, and caught the contrary wind full on.

The ship lurched, listed dangerously, righted, and careened around broadside to the wind. When Atawulf saw the wave billowing toward them he scarcely had time to shout a warning.

A surge of water lifted the vessel, canted it sideways, tossed it high on the swell, and dropped it into the trough behind. The ship groaned and wallowed; horses stumbled and screamed; Atawulf saw one of his men plummet into the sea.

Close upon the first wave, another struck the floundering ship. Blinding torrents of seawater rained upon their heads, washed the deck, and dragged at the boat, nearly overturning it. But the craft was seaworthy and bobbed back up, flinging spray and men across the decks. Above the shriek of wind came a screaming, shouting chaos from below decks, along with the panicked kicks and screams of horses.

As they rode atop a surge of waves, Atawulf's eyes met the horrifying sight of at least one ship down, rolling helplessly in the water, already half-swallowed by the wild sea.

He had only time for a glance, for now his own ship spun about in a whirlwind which circled and howled like squalling, spitting cats, and Atawulf saw a new disaster awaiting them. As the storm increased, wave upon wave bore upon them, driving them recklessly, relentlessly toward a jagged line of rocks which jutted into the strait as though to catch them in their stormswept flight.

"Drop your armor!" screamed Atawulf into the howling wind, but the words were hurled back down his throat. Shouting was futile amid the furious snapping of sails, the shrill singing of the wind, the roar and splash of great waves which spilled over the sides of the crazily pitching vessel.

He tore at the bucklings of his own breastplate and sent it hurtling into the sea. Some of the men, looking toward their commander for a miracle, saw Atawulf throw off his armor and they followed his lead, unbuckling breastplates and swordbelts, tossing aside helmets. Every man pouring up from the bowels of the ship did the same, for any moment the spinning ship must rip to pieces upon the breakers, and a hard, wild sea foamed between the jagged line of rocks and the craggy shore.

Atawulf pulled himself along a line of rigging and stumbled down the loading ramp to reach the horses, who were tied head to head one deck below, a deck now awash with water knee-deep.

He reached the lead horse first, his own Red Demon. He drew his dagger and cut Demon's cinch, letting the saddle fall. Then he laid a steadying hand on his war-horse's heaving side, stroked the jerking head, and cut the reins which held the animal. He let Demon go and began working his way down the line of horses, relieved to see that several of his horse soldiers had followed and come to his aid in releasing the confined horses. Above, more men had the presence of mind to shove open the large loading hatches so that at least some of the horses might have a chance of escaping a dreadful drowning trapped in the dark hold.

Of a sudden there came a lull in the storm. The wind seemed almost to die, the sea churned in confusion, the ship sheeted about again only to meet a fresh fury. As Atawulf struggled up the ramp, a tremendous crack overhead made him look up to see the topmast snap and fall, the sharp sharded end hanging dangerously, caught in the rigging. The topsail collapsed, blanketing the men on the forward deck.

Now, despairingly, Atawulf saw the great wave, high as a mountain, surging upon them and cresting to terrifying height over what was left of the mast. The monstrous wave broke clean across the beam of the ship and rolled the craft with it in the tremendous curve of its descent, overthrowing men and horses as it deluged the decks in a pounding torrent.

No chance to pray, just hold on for life. Atawulf's fingers and arms ached from clinging to the stump of the mast. The sea descended upon his head, filled his eyes and mouth, and every gasping breath seemed a lungful of salt water.

Before the ship could overturn, he felt a wrenching shock as the hull struck an underwater rock and dragged across it. The whole vessel shuddered, planking splintered, and the sea poured into the rupture.

The backwash of the wave stranded the vessel half on its side atop the underwater breaker, but only for a breath-catching instant, for a whole mountain range of waves rose from the raging sea, frothing and gnashing and racing to their destruction.

The next breaking wave struck with such ferocity it blasted them free, but drove them rapidly toward the craggy headlands. The ship rode low, struck an underwater shelf, and dragged across it.

With a sickening crunch the sea dashed the ship onto jagged rocks. The abrupt collision and the steep slant of the ship sent frantic horses plunging through a rent in the hull and into the foaming hazard. The keel broke, the bow shattered and drove upward, forcing the forward third of the ship into a fissure between two outcroppings. The forward deck, with its canopy of torn sail, collapsed amidships, raining splintered fragments onto the few horses still trapped below decks. The unfortunate creatures screamed in fear and pain as the ship buckled in upon them.

As the sea washed up over the wedged ship, Atawulf heard screams and pleas for help from men entangled in the fallen rigging. The agonized cries and entreaties from those wounded and those pinned down in the wreckage of the rigging, spars, and sails drew Atawulf and others to scramble forward to free them.

One man, and Atawulf knew him, lay pierced through by a

broken spar, writhing in agony, blood gurgling from his throat as he tried to scream.

As swiftly as they leapt to the aid of their companions, the sea was swifter. Another huge wave slammed into the ship, beating it ferociously against the crags, and with a tremendous shudder and deep groan like that of a wounded beast, the vessel gave up the fight and burst asunder; the midsection, with its dreadful cargo of trapped men and horses, grated slowly down the ragged rocks.

Atawulf and the clinging men were forced to leap for the rocks, while behind them the pitiful cries of the doomed were gradually silenced beneath the churning sea.

The survivors scrambled up slippery shards of rock, clinging with bloodied hands when the next wave washed over them, tugging at them tirelessly to fling them back into the sea. But they were climbing the craggy feet of the cliff; above them a rise of dark boulders glittered in the spray, higher than the relentless waves.

Then another crippled vessel dashed broadside upon the wreck of the first. Atawulf strained to see through the spray and hovering mist flung up by crashing waves, for he thought it was Alaric's ship. He found Alaric aboard the wreckage, his foster brother's powerful shoulders straining as he held to the railing near the bow. Only one hand gripped the rail; the other hauled one of his men back up over the side, but even as the man reached safety, the bow tipped, a boom swung wild and struck Alaric in the back of the head. Alaric fell like a stone into the sea.

Atawulf stared in horror at the frothy surface where Alaric disappeared. Sucking in a huge breath, Atawulf hurled himself into the air, plunged feet first into the sea just where the foam had closed over Alaric's head.

He shot downward like an arrow loosed from a bow, sinking faster than the limp form of Alaric. Forcing his eyes open in the brackish, foaming turbulence, he thought a black form tumbled nearby. He kicked for it, grasped it, knew it was human. Desperate, with all the will and muscle in his limbs, he pulled toward the surface.

Air and sky seemed a lifetime away, but at last, when his head broke from the churning sea into blessed salt-laden air, he gasped and sucked in wind and sea-spray.

He had only a moment to grab another breath, but it was enough to assure him it was Alaric he held—Alaric, floating senseless and weighing heavy in his arms—before yet another wave bore them down.

The backlash had pulled them farther out to sea, but now the capricious waves swept them toward the craggy shore again with terrifying speed. Underwater Atawulf held on to Alaric and braced both feet out before him, braced for a smash upon jagged rocks. By luck or divine aid his feet struck the submerged rock first, and they skittered around it. When at last they surfaced, they were in an eddy between boulders.

Atawulf's burning lungs fought for breath; a floating section of planking struck the side of his head. He grabbed for it, slipped, grabbed again and found a handhold in a ragged piece of hull. Then they were dragged from the eddy back into the full fury of the waves.

He fought to cling to the planking, to keep them both afloat. Holding Alaric pinned against him, his right arm across Alaric's chest, he gripped his fingers tightly in the leather jerkin under Alaric's arm. His left arm stretched across the plank, where he held to a jagged tear in the wood, and Atawulf could do naught but hold on with all his strength as the sea tossed them wildly.

He saw the mountain of water rising impossibly, like something out of nightmare, higher and higher; he saw it peak and begin to curl, and Bold Wolf knew it would sunder his one-handed grip on Alaric. He let go of the planking, threw both arms around Alaric's lifeless body, gasped and closed his eyes as the wave crested, spilled, and pounded them downward.

The unbearable weight of water drove them deep. Lungs near bursting, Atawulf felt his feet hit solid bottom, and he shoved off, straight up, with every bit of strength in his legs.

They surfaced in the wake of the wave, drawn again away

from shore and out to sea. And the sea seemed determined to swallow them. Atawulf choked on salt water; his leggings clung and dragged at him like leaden chains, and every second was an agony of fatigue.

Bold Wolf fought the fiercest, most terrifying and deadly foe of his life, and for the first time he felt defeat, death's cold maw opening to swallow him, the sucking sea dragging him down—and he fought all the harder. He would have screamed defiance at the waves if he had breath or strength.

His mind centered on one thought: hold on. If Alaric went down, Atawulf would go down with him.

Around him in the water collided the wreckage and fragments of shattered vessels. A spar bobbed nearby, and Atawulf pulled toward it. Wrapping his left arm over the spar, he rested his legs for a blessed moment. Fighting for breath, he looked wildly about for shore—a jagged wall of black—and seawater filled his eyes and nostrils and throat as another wave sped them forward, straight for that jagged wall.

Rolling beneath them, the wave dropped them into its trough—like dropping down a precipice, it felt, and Atawulf hung on to that spar and to Alaric with single-minded, ferocious devotion. His arms and shoulders burned with the exertion, his muscles cramped, shrieking to be released, and his legs, numb and leaden, barely responded to his will.

The next wave lifted and carried them on toward the jagged boulders and clefts with a force that could but dash them mercilessly on the rocks. Then the spar hit something, jammed, and snapped in two. Atawulf and Alaric were flung between the deadly outcroppings; they went under and struck a hard surface; Atawulf's left arm and shoulder took the blow. All nerve and feeling left him, and he knew he must have lost Alaric. When his head cleared the water, his lungs heaving, Atawulf found his body would not respond. The sea dragged him down, his head sinking beneath the waves.

Suddenly hands grasped the neck of his jerkin, fingers hooked under his arm, and he was being pulled up on the rocks. His burning eyes saw hazily through a glassy film of pain.

Men were in the sea and on the rocks, reaching with strong arms to pull him from the water. Wallia and others had hold of him—and Alaric, for he had not lost his grip on him after all—and the rescuers grasped them firmly as waves spilled over their heads. Slowly, painstakingly, they brought Atawulf and Alaric to the top of the cleft into which they had been washed by the sea.

Atawulf lay on his back and sucked grateful gulps of air, having somehow signaled to Wallia that he was all right. Desperate activity, frantic and dismayed curses, clamored beside him, and he knew the men were trying to save Alaric.

Slowly, excruciating fire searing through his left shoulder and arm, Atawulf managed to turn on his right side and blink burning eyes, bringing the tense knot of men into focus. They gathered about Alaric's limp form, shaking him, calling him, trying to support the lolling head of their chief, their king.

A freed Saxon arrived, breathless, claiming he grew up with the sea and had seen men revived when all believed them drowned. He bade them roll Alaric onto his stomach, and he straddled the lifeless body of the man who had always been so full of motion and energy and strength that they could scarcely comprehend this unresponding, moveless flesh. The Saxon, with strong, broad hands, pressed and pressed and pressed, as though he flattened bread, while the silent circle of Goths stood or squatted and watched with grave faces.

Atawulf saw Winnifreya struggle across the rocks, followed by a score of women. His vision blurred as his sister bent over him, though whether it was from injury or grief he did not know. She touched his shoulder and he winced from the fire of it; she jerked her hand away, then gently touched his face. Now she turned her head, her fair face colorless with shock, and watched the Saxon pounding on her husband's still form.

A whimper lodged in her throat, and Atawulf moved his right hand to touch hers. Brother and sister locked fingers while the man they both loved lay lifeless beneath the determined hands of the Saxon.

They did not truly expect it, but the miracle happened. Suddenly Alaric gagged and vomited seawater. He choked, heaved, spewed water, and dragged at a breath which rattled in his chest and caused him to choke again. More water came up, and more and more from his stomach and lungs, but Alaric was gagging and fighting and, Father in Heaven, *breathing*.

The Saxon rolled off Alaric with a grin as wide as the sky, and Wallia grabbed the man and hugged him, so inexpressible was his gratitude. Winnifreya flew to her husband's side, heedless of the vomit and phlegm smeared over his face and hair.

Atawulf sighed and closed his eyes. Alaric was alive, not drowned in the cold, raging sea. Though Atawulf could hear roaring surf and growling thunder, though a steady rain pelted him, it all seemed very far away, and he was sinking into a black sea of his own, but this time he need not fight it; he had won his battle. He had wrested his brother from the sea, and he did not fear to let the black night close over his head.

Dia did not remember leaving the terrace; she scarcely recalled running along the beach with the others, though she surely had, for here she stood in pouring rain on the rocky bluff, clutching her cloak in tight fists. She had only been aware that Atawulf's ship was rolling and breaking and smashing upon the rocks and that she must, somehow, get to him.

Now Winnifreya had gone to Alaric, and Atawulf lay alone, his face etched with pain. Dia approached him softly, knelt, and placed a trembling hand upon his cold, wet brow. He groaned, but his eyes remained closed.

Dia had not known her heart could feel so much pain and joy in one instant. Pain to see him so injured, joy to know he still lived.

"Bold Wolf," she whispered, her voice barely audible above the rain. "My dear, brave Bold Wolf."

Was it in her imagination that a smile seemed to flicker briefly on his lips? Certainly he stirred. Then Singledia the Elder knelt at her side, summoning help for her son.

"Lift him gently, now," Singledia ordered. "Get him out of the rain so I can find where he's hurt."

Two Goths labored to raise Atawulf to a sitting position. He cried out in pain and shoved at them with his uninjured arm. Now more cautiously they helped him to his feet, but when they tried to lead him away from the cliff, he shook his head and stared into the strait, stared at the wreckage of ships upon the breakers and jagged rocks. Men still struggled in the turbulent water between the line of breakers and the boulders and clefts of the mainland.

"Help those men up the rocks!" Atawulf bellowed, turning to descend the bluff himself to reach the water's edge. His mother tried to stop him, but he shook her off. Then he came face to face with Dia, who put out her hands to halt this foolhardy disregard of his injury.

"Atawulf . . ."

His stare was bleak. "I hope you're satisfied."

"What? I don't—"

"This is what you prayed for, isn't it? The destruction of our plans, the end of the Goths?"

"No, I—"

"Well, you got what you wanted, nobilissima. Enjoying it?"

Dia stood speechless as he brushed past her. What was he saying? How could he accuse her of praying for this? His cruel words cut to her very soul, and the whole world seemed to stop around her as she stood frozen. Scarcely noticing the wind-blown rain that soaked her, she turned and watched him descend the bluff unsteadily, supported by one of the warriors.

She felt she might die of a burst heart on the spot. A long time she stood there, unmoving, long after Atawulf passed from her sight, until Singledia put a strong arm around her and turned her away with gentle words.

"Don't take it to heart, Placidia. We all know prayers of yours did not cause this destruction. Atawulf knows it, and he'll realize it when he comes to himself."

Dia drew in a shuddering breath and shook her head, unable to speak, or she would have told the mother of Atawulf that he had meant what he said; he believed a monstrous thing of her, and furthermore, he wanted to believe it, for he had not bothered to hear her protests, had not wanted to know the truth.

She was glad of the rain, at least, so that none could see the flood of tears that streamed down her icy cheeks.

Weary to the bone, Atawulf stood on the ragged beach and watched the rescuers struggle up from the water's edge. There had been survivors—men and a few horses—but the toll on life, so sudden and savage, was unbearable to contemplate.

Now that the storm had died down to a brisk cold wind, the tide slipped back and left the shore littered with wreckage. Fragments of the shattered flotilla washed in from the breakers, floated against the cliffs. The few vessels which had still been in the harbor, or close enough to reach it, were still afloat, but many of those in the middle of the strait had capsized and sunk, taking their passengers down with them.

The rest were crippled on the breakers or shredded into miles of debris.

Atawulf closed his eyes against the scene, for washing into shore like part of the wreckage were the broken bodies of men and horses, beaten against the cruel rocks. Some of the faces of the men were unrecognizable, but he knew them—he had known them all his life.

Fully two-thirds of the men who set out had perished, and nearly all the horses.

Atawulf, desolate and angry, stared at the sea, the impervious sea, rolling untroubled and untouched toward him, throwing spray and mist up the cliffs, mindlessly pounding its terrible carnage over and over against the jagged rocks.

Atawulf swallowed hard, willing his grief to turn to rage. God, he hated the sea. He hated this accursed shore, this inhospitable country at the end of the world, and he hated this Empire which swallowed up the Earth and gave none of it back, which made no free people welcome unless they bent their backs and became its slaves. He hated Rome and its Emperor and all Romans—even *her,* he even hated her because she was Rome, Rome and all it stood for.

His dry eyes stung with pain, but he kept them open to the horror and the loss. His arm and shoulder, his whole left side, throbbed with agony, but he could not bring himself to leave the wretched shore. He could not abandon the dead. He had ordered the men and women to rest before taking on the grim task of pulling bodies out of the sea. They had resisted; many of them still wandered up and down the beach in grief, searching for bodies of loved ones. Nor could Atawulf rest. He felt he could never rest again. He would never close his eyes again without seeing what he saw now, so he simply stared.

So dark and inward was his vision that for some moments he didn't see the distant shape struggling down the beach. Then he squinted in the late-afternoon light muted by grey clouds racing after the storm.

A horse slowly walked a cautious path among the boulders from which the storm-tide had receded. Atawulf thought it stumbled. The horse's head drooped, but when Atawulf moved toward it, the head lifted, red face and mane ruddy in the hazy light, a streak of white between the eyes.

Demon.

Atawulf quickened his steps, heedless of the pain in his side. Demon. He almost feared to believe it.

The red stallion waited for him, too weary to move, but his ears flicked forward.

"Demon!"

A low whicker, fading into an almost human sigh, greeted him.

The horse's legs trembled, and his shins were red and raw from scraping on the rocks. Gashes crisscrossed his flanks, and the bedraggled mane was plastered to his neck with salt and blood.

But Red Demon watched him coming with eyes soft and clear. Atawulf touched the trembling horse, and the noble head dropped for sympathy.

"Demon, you made it," Atawulf murmured, his voice thick with amazement and relief. One arm pressed around the horse's neck, he buried his face in the salty coat.

"I made it, too," he whispered, and then he wept.

In dazed grief, the Goths buried their dead. Others they lamented, but could not bury, those whose bodies lay trapped in sunken hulks or drifted along the bottom of the strait. The Goths, in their devastation, seldom spoke as they went about the task of digging graves and laying beloved husbands, fathers, sons, and brothers to rest.

Their shock ran deep, and words, words were nothing. Pain and loss were all, and when words were spoken they returned always to the same question, like stones falling down a well. *Why?*

The Roman populace of Rhegium stood aside and watched the Goths with faces grave and wary. Even they were subdued by the magnitude of the disaster. The Daughters of Rhea, those peasant women and girls who had danced under the solstice stars and called on the help of the Mother Goddess, even they looked upon the Goths with awe and pity, for they had never seen any folk so suffer the wrath of wind and sea, and it would be many a year before they again dared curse their enemies with the power of the Mother.

In the churches, the priests held forth on the tragedy of the Goths. This was what came of heresy and savagery. The Lord God would not countenance it; he destroyed the Goths as he destroyed the armies of the Pharaoh at Moses's command. The priests led the people in prayer, thanking God for taking their side, the side of righteousness, and for breaking the will of the foe.

It was true; the will of the Goths was broken. Their proud spirits were broken; grief weighed down their hearts and minds and slowed their steps. Their road ended here, at the hard toe of the peninsula. Even could they assemble another fleet, not a man, woman, or child among them had the courage to set out to sea. Their hearts and minds were too filled with the terrible tragedy they had witnessed.

Atawulf didn't blame them. The sea was their enemy, in his mind, as much as Rome was their enemy. Alaric himself could not have ordered the Bold Wolf to attempt another crossing.

Not that Alaric would, Atawulf thought grimly. Alaric had not ordered anything in two days. He sank back into the fever from which he had been recovering, the near drowning seeming to weaken his body and give the fever new strength. The king came before his people but once, to see the many graves they filled with the broken remains of his proud warriors.

"We cannot stay here," Atawulf told Alaric as his brother lay in a house confiscated for his recovery. "There are not enough winter stores to feed us. We have no choice but to continue along the coast, which I am loath to do, or return the way we came until we reach the inland highway. Our people want no more to do with the sea, nor do I."

Alaric closed his eyes as though his brother's words were a torment.

"Which do you want us to do, Alaric?"

"You choose," Alaric whispered, his throat rattling a little with each shallow breath.

"I say we retreat and then cut inland." *Retreat*, Atawulf thought bitterly as he said the word. Just as she said we would have to do. He thrust her from his thoughts and concentrated on Alaric.

"Do you think you can travel?"

"I'll travel." Alaric reached up and caught Atawulf's uninjured hand. "I'm sorry."

Atawulf shook his head. "Sorry for what? That you're ill? That a storm overtook us? Which of these is your fault?"

"I brought us here."

"You couldn't have known." When Alaric made no answer, Atawulf spoke gently. "If it was the wrong course, then we'll try another one."

Alaric closed his eyes. His words were faint and struggling. "Too late. Too late for the men who drowned, too late for their families. I failed them, Atawulf. I failed my people."

Atawulf looked to Winnifreya, who sat nearby. Tears welled in her eyes, and the helpless, stricken grief in her face cut him to the quick. He turned back to Alaric, gripping his hot hand. Sweat beaded on Alaric's brow, dampened his hair and the pillows on which he was propped to ease his breathing.

"That's fever talking, brother. You haven't failed any of us. When you've recovered 'twill all look different."

Agitated, Alaric rolled his head from side to side. "You don't see. I pitted myself against Rome . . . for pride . . . for revenge . . . and I brought death on my people. Even God turned against us . . . sent a storm to destroy us." His blue eyes, too bright, brilliant with fever, met Atawulf's with despair and defeat, and his voice sank. "Rome wins . . . and God abandons us at the end of the Earth. Tell them . . . ask them . . . to forgive me."

Atawulf fought for his voice.

"No need, Alaric," he said roughly. "They forgive you. And we are not lost." He attempted a careless grin, but it felt more like a grimace of pain. "The Romans don't have us yet, brother, and I know you. The fight's not out of you; you'll be up and making life hell for the Emperor again."

But even as he spoke those words, Atawulf knew they were useless.

Alaric knew it, too. He dropped his head back, tormented by fever and his panting struggle for breath. He had not even the strength or will to reply. Winnifreya bent over him, bathing his flushed face with a cloth dipped in cool water. When she looked toward Atawulf across Alaric's burning body, her eyes were sunken with sleeplessness and worry. She shook her head, warning her brother to speak no more to him.

Atawulf nodded, swallowing his grief, and sat in silence, watching his sister bathe her husband's forehead, his face and neck, his broad shoulders and chest, and it hardly seemed possible that Alaric, always so strong, so invincible, should be helpless in the grip of fever and despair.

He stayed until the physician returned, waving the man away when he would check his own bandaged arm and shoulder, and stayed long enough to watch the concocting of a steam of hyssop, willow, and fennel and the mixing of a bitter tea of absinth and willow bark, in hopes of bringing Alaric's fever down. When he left the hot, stuffy sickroom, Bold Wolf breathed in great lungfuls of cool sea air, but it was air he hated, this salt-tang bitter on his tongue.

Had he not known how useless it was, Atawulf would have cursed God and Heaven and Hell for what they had done to Alaric—not so much for laying him low with fever, but for dealing him such a blow of defeat, for tearing the hope and spirit out of him just when Alaric needed them the most. But Atawulf was not given to useless railings at fate or chance. He shifted his bound arm with a groan, trying to ease the pain in his shoulder, and sucked in another great breath, knowing what happened now was up to him, at least as long as Alaric was ill. And Atawulf had already chosen his course.

The Goths would return as rapidly as they could up the coast whence they had come. In a few days they would reach a branching where the highway divided. Via Appia, the highway they had traveled south from Rome, followed the coast. But Via Popilia turned inland, running northward up the peninsula, leading straight through the mountainous heartland of Italia. Atawulf had questioned countless people about this road; the farther north they traveled, the more fertile and productive would be the land, which meant a greater abundance of food for the Goths.

Atawulf wished to reach the branching of the highway quickly, for though he had heard everything to the contrary, he found it hard to believe that Ravenna would not be sending legions to cut them off. Had he been Emperor, he would have done so long ago. Could Honorius truly be such a fool, such a poor general? Were his advisors also the stupidest men on the face of the Earth? Or were they simply sacrificing their own people, sitting safe behind the marshes, letting the Goths wear themselves out seeking escape from the dead end they had reached?

Forgetting how much pain sudden motion would cause him, he shook himself, not willing to complete that thought. No, he told himself, there would be no legions meeting them upon the highway. For one thing, word could not possibly reach Ravenna of the Goths' disaster soon enough for Honorius to seize his advantage. By then, the Goths would be deep in the forests and hills, where the advantage would be theirs.

Atawulf found it hard to believe that the present Emperor could have come from the loins of Theodosius. Old Theo would have surrounded them at Rome the first time they laid siege to the city, just as Dia claimed *she* would have done. Aye, hard to believe Honorius shared the same blood as Galla Placidia, even by half. What an implacable enemy she would make if the power of an Emperor were hers.

Even now she was probably thanking God for their destruction and for the death of so many fighting men and horses. Oh, aye, she was Roman and she had made it clear what she thought of the Goths and where her loyalty lay. And what did he expect?

Atawulf ground his teeth. How in blazes had he let himself forget who and what she was? The pain he felt over her hatred of his people was all the worse because he knew he had been a fool for letting her get under his skin. Well, he had come to his senses now. Bold Wolf knew where his loyalty belonged, and Galla Placidia could never be anything but his enemy.

Dia leaned back on the driver's bench of the coach as if she were checking the stars for direction, but the coach sat still, having been unhitched for the night. Thalia climbed up beside her. The two of them had come out in their warm wraps to enjoy the cool night breeze.

"He doesn't speak to me," Dia continued as Thalia settled. "And if he is *forced* to ride past, why, he doesn't even look in our direction."

"I know."

"It's like he's punishing me. And I didn't just order up some storm from God like . . . like God was my . . . my Master of Offices or something."

"No, of course not. And he doesn't believe that, either."

"No, he's punishing me for what he *thinks* I prayed for that night." Dia gave a little laugh, half-irony, half-despair. "I swear, Thalia, I never once prayed for harm to come to his people."

"I know. You've sworn it a dozen times, and I believe you. Why don't you swear it to him?"

Still leaning back on the bench, Dia turned her head to look indignantly at Thalia.

"You mean *defend* myself? Certainly not." She glared straight up at the stars again.

"Oh. How silly of me," said Thalia a little sullenly. "What an unreasonable notion."

Dia sat up and turned to face her. "Absolutely unreasonable. See here, Thalia, I have done nothing wrong. *He's* the one who's jumped to conclusions about what's going on in *my* mind. Why, the very idea that I should have to defend myself over something which is entirely in his imagination! I'll not stoop to giving credence to his horrible, hateful accusations!"

By now her words had exploded into bursts of anger, just at the edge of tears, but she caught a deep breath, blinked hard, and glared at the swimming stars. She refused to cry, to acknowledge how much it hurt that he believed the worst of her. He said cruel things to her, things of which she was innocent, and it did not seem fair that she should be the one feeling hurt and miserable.

"How will he ever know he's wrong if no one tells him?"

"Tell him? Let him suffer until he figures it out."

"Seems to me, he's not the only one suffering, mistress."

Dia propped her arms on her knees and cradled her head in them. The worst of it was, she couldn't deny that it mattered very much to her what Atawulf thought.

And how could she be feeling this impossible turmoil: hating Atawulf for his accusation in one moment, her heart aching for his grief the next moment? She wanted to go to him, comfort him, but she knew she would be rebuffed, and her hurt was too great for that. She was not that brave.

Thalia, acutely aware of her mistress's distress, said gently, "Suppose *I* went to Atawulf, and told him the truth myself?"

Without raising her head, Dia shook it from side to side. "If you go, it will be the same as if I went to him. Don't you see, he'd be sure I sent you."

Thalia was indignant. "It was my idea. I'd be going on my own."

"He'd never believe that." Dia raised her head and stared at her maid suspiciously. "Thalia, I simply forbid you to do any such thing. You will not say one word to Atawulf. I will not be humiliated."

"Yes, miss," Thalia said quietly, folding her hands and staring at them in the dark. She knew from Dia's sharp tone that argument would be worse than futile—the Imperial Princess would become furiously adamant and all possibility of changing her mind would be ruined.

They stared silently at the stars until Dia decided the air was too cool and the sky too oppressively *vast* for sitting out, and they went in to bed.

Atawulf did not rest easily until the Gothic caravan reached the split in the highway and left the coast behind. He pushed them and pushed himself, never resting enough, never giving the pain in his shoulder and arm time to let up. The sea made him uneasy; its constant surging seemed to taunt him with the deaths of his men, and he felt trapped with the expanse of water always cutting off retreat in the west.

Now, as the inland highway climbed steadily into hilly country, he felt in his element again—hilltops to fortify, high ground to climb and watch for any movement of legions. The scouts reported none.

The Goths traveled with grieving hearts and empty bellies. The route they retraced held no sustenance for them, for they had already plundered the coast for its food supplies; foraging parties searched now for winter stores in this rugged inland country. Atawulf kept the people moving, feeling some disaster was about to overtake them, though he knew the disaster he most feared could never be outrun.

Alaric was dying.

Though Atawulf's heart denied it, his mind knew it. Alaric's fever burned day and night, and he had to be always propped upright or the breath rattled like death in his throat. And now he coughed up blood.

Alaric, dying. To Atawulf the very thought was a nightmare, and he kept expecting to awaken and discover his brother, his friend, recovered and grinning at him hugely. But the defeated looks on the physicians' faces and the weary terror in Winnifreya's eyes told him this was real.

Alaric, dying.

Atawulf hesitated before the wagon which carried Alaric, reluctant to enter. His mother had found him and told him he should come as soon as possible. "Alaric needs to speak with you," Singledia had said, but it was the urgent gravity in her voice that drew him here quickly.

Atawulf squared his shoulders, painfully, and pushed aside the wagon's oxhide covering. His heart sank further as he saw that one of the occupants of the wagon was Bishop Sigesarius.

Atawulf pulled himself one-handed into the wagon, which stank of sickness, and approached the figure leaning upon a prop of pillows and blankets. The blue eyes which met his were dull and feverish, sunken in dark hollows, and the face from which they stared was sallow and sickly. The Alaric he knew, so full of strength and vitality, was shrunken and too weak to sit up on his own.

The wagon's interior seemed filled with the sound of horrendously painful breathing, every lungful of air a struggle to the death, but Alaric's cracked lips moved in silent greeting to his brother.

"Alaric," said Bold Wolf huskily, his voice sounding in his ears too deep and robust in the presence of this breath-stealing fever. He sat beside the bed on a stool that Winnifreya vacated for him.

For a while Alaric did not speak; he seemed to be gathering strength, so Atawulf told him how the camp fared, neglecting to mention they had found no new food in four days. When Atawulf fell into silence, Alaric laid a hand on his and began to speak—a long, laborious process which pained those who listened almost as much as it pained Alaric.

"You," the ragged words began, "you will take my place . . . lead the people . . . I choose . . . you."

"Aye, brother, until you are well."

Atawulf waved an impatient hand at him. "I choose Atawulf . . . King." The sunken eyes looked to Bishop Sigesarius demandingly. "Be my witness." Then, to his wife, "You, too . . . Winn. Atawulf must lead . . . stand together."

Winnifreya nodded, tears filling her eyes.

Again Alaric looked to Atawulf, reaching for him. Atawulf caught his brother's hand and held it tightly.

"I failed." When Atawulf tried to object, Alaric shook his head weakly. "I'm tired, brother . . . you do better . . . take them . . . find them a home . . ."

Atawulf bowed his head, tears running freely. "I will," he told his brother hoarsely.

"Good . . ."

"You didn't fail us, Alaric! We are not lost, and Rome has not won." His words were fierce. "We are still free! You've fed us and clothed us and given us victory over our enemies!"

Alaric's crusted lips tried to smile. "Now you give them . . . what you wanted . . . you give them . . . peace."

Atawulf's lips pressed together in a hard line. There could never be peace with Rome, not now, not after the Empire had broken Alaric's spirit, but he nodded once, jerkily, and gripped the dry, slack hand in his.

Alaric tried to say more, but he gasped for breath and was racked with a fit of coughing—painful, rasping coughs that strove to clear his lungs—but nothing loosened in his heaving chest, and the spasm left him sucking the air like a drowning man desperate to breathe. Atawulf had the terrible notion that the sea from which he rescued his brother had lurked in his lungs and lain in wait and now gurgled up from the inside to drown him.

Like an icy hand clamping the back of his neck, horror laid hold of him. His brother and king was dying, wrenching out one resisting breath at a time, knowing each one might be the last, but willing it not to be this one. The sea would have him after all, mocking, laughing at Atawulf's puny effort to save him. Never before had Atawulf felt so defeated—and he hated it, just as he hated the sea and the Empire.

Alaric, dying.

Atawulf saw Alaric quietened, saw Winnifreya bathe his face and wet his lips with cool water, saw the glazed blue eyes close and clench with the struggle to live, and he departed the wagon to the sound of the bishop murmuring softly. Outside he stood in the afternoon shadows and wept, the tears drying cold on his face and beard.

Late in the night Alaric lost his battle. Death wrested the last rattling breath from him and left him silent and still and empty.

Winnifreya bowed her head upon Alaric's unresponsive shoulder and shook with sobs so deep and agonizing they could not be released, just held in her gut, shuddering, beating her from the inside, but she would not let them go, as if by holding them back she could hold on to Alaric just a little longer.

The mourning Goths seemed all the more terrible to Dia because they mourned in knots of silence. Tears streamed soundlessly down faces listless, grim, or fearful. All the day before they had streamed past the wooden bier on which the body of their valiant king and chieftain lay composed and arrayed in a war chief's splendor. This morning they would bury him with the full honors due a barbarian king.

"He is the greatest of our warriors," Atawulf had told them, "the greatest of our chieftains, and the first and best King of the Goths. Alaric will be buried as the chiefs of old."

Therefore this morning Dia stood to one side as the Goths prepared to bury their king. She felt more distant from the Goths at this moment than any since she had been their captive. Their grief was like a grey wall around them, shutting her out of their hearts and minds. Though she was surprised to find herself grieving for the arrogant, mocking Alaric—somehow she had grown to like him in these few months—she could never feel the depth of loss or anguish that the Gothic people felt.

Their beloved Alaric dead, never again to goad them, cajole

them, reassure them, laugh with them, brighten the very air about him with his sure and shining presence.

But the grief Dia felt for those who loved Alaric most was keen and deep. She knew the soul-wrenching pain of losing someone dear and beloved, and her heart went out to Winnifreya who loved him, to the daughters who adored him, and Singledia who had raised him as her own, and to Atawulf who could neither remember nor imagine a lifetime without the constant, easy companionship of his brother and friend.

Oh, yes, especially Atawulf. Dia ached for him the most.

She watched him now, walking slowly toward where Alaric lay. Atawulf looked as barbaric as the Goths of old who had never set foot on Roman soil. He wore rough hide breeches and vest, his sword belted on with gem-inlaid, tooled leather. His beard was split into six stiff braids twisted with red leather, and two thick ropes of yellow hair hung on either side of his face, while the rest of his hair fell loose and wild. In addition to armbands and wristbands inlaid with lapis and garnet, he wore a heavy torque of twisted gold at his throat.

A ragged, musty, black wolf's head with carnelian eyes glared from atop his head, the shaggy black pelt trailing down his back and shoulders. And on his right arm, the arm not strapped tight to his side with linen bandaging, on his free arm he carried an old round shield with a black grinning wolf painted on the rawhide surface.

Atawulf. Bold Wolf.

But most of all Dia saw his eyes.

They were dark bruises of agony, and his face was drawn around them in deep gashes of pain. Those eyes saw nothing but the shell of Alaric, fixed on nothing but what they had lost.

Dia's heart wept for him, and forgetting her indignant little tirade of days ago—as Thalia knew she would—she felt the pull of his grief, left the little knoll on which she stood, and approached him with open hands and open heart.

"Atawulf," she murmured softly. "I'm so sorry . . ."

He stopped, but he scarcely seemed to see her. In his dark, hollow eyes was room for nothing but wrenching agony.

"So sorry," she said. "I know you loved him . . . your brother."

Those terrible, haunted eyes stared at her, and something hard and angry glittered in their blue depths.

"Aye," he muttered darkly. "I know how sorry you are—Roman."

Half-angered herself, half-grieved, her words were low and resonant as she sought reason. "Surely you know I never wished harm to Alaric, nor any of your people. If you believe I rejoice over this, you're a fool."

The pain and rage in those eyes were impenetrable. The rage, for all it may have been rage at Fate or God, turned full on her, for Fate and God were out of his reach and Galla Placidia stood before him, challenging his hate with that stubborn purpose in the set of her mouth, the low pitch of determination in her voice.

"Step aside, Roman," he gritted at her. "You are not welcome here."

She saw that, clearly. Slowly, without taking her gaze from his, she picked the hem of her cloak out of the dust and stepped aside. Atawulf strode past her brusquely, his terrible eyes seeking the death bier of Alaric and seeing none else.

Dia felt her heart wrench, for Atawulf and his grief, for herself and her inability to reach him, but she knew this was nothing to the wound in Atawulf's heart. Defeated, she climbed the sloping ground to where Thalia and Priscus Attalus waited, outsiders here. Even Attalus had no part in this farewell to Alaric, King of the Goths, but the old statesman's eyes swam with sorrow as he watched the procession of mourners approach and encircle the lonely bier.

Alaric lay in kingly splendor upon the wooden platform. He was arrayed in a cloak of crimson wool trimmed with gold-thread embroidery, fastened at one shoulder by an intricate brooch inlaid with a swirled design. His boots were of red leather, and on his brow they had placed a heavy circlet of gold inlaid with garnet, lapis, and jet.

About his neck he wore a torque of twisted gold fashioned into two lions' heads facing each other at his throat. A massive belt buckle of rich and intricate design held the belt about his raw-leather vest. And on his bare arms, once so inflamed with life, now so still and cold, were set armbands and wristbands and rings of garnet and lapis, amber, jet, and amethyst.

Beside him rested two swords, sheathed in finely tooled leather, with richly ornate hilts, and with them a javelin. At his feet lay a shield, iron embossed with bronze, and a saddle and horse harness of red leather.

Bishop Sigesarius stepped slowly forward and fastened around Alaric's neck a chain and laid upon his breast a gold disk monogrammed with a Chi-Rho in red and blue enamel.

But it was when Winnifreya knelt on the ground beside the body of her husband that Dia thought her heart would break. The queen slipped a ring from her finger and gently worked it onto Alaric's little finger, then she kissed the pale brow.

Now she slid the jeweled dagger from Alaric's belt and flung back the blue veil that covered her hair. Head back, eyes to the heavens, she gripped the hilt, raised her arms, and sheared off her single long golden braid.

Longingly, she coiled the braid beneath his right hand, and as she bowed her head to this last, dread task, the nape of her neck bare, cropped hair shining in the sun, Dia for the first time saw how fragile looked the Queen of the Goths, fragile and lost.

Her hand trembling, Winnifreya passed the dagger on to her daughters, who, with tears streaking their faces, imitated their mother and cut off their own braids. They twined the braids together to lay with their mother's beneath their father's hand. Singledia the Elder joined them, adding her own grey hair to her foster son's bier.

Atawulf stood long and looked at the shrunken figure on the bier. The Alaric he knew was no more. That pathetic form told Atawulf the truth most plainly, and he found he could not bear to look any longer. He signaled the waiting wagon to be driven forth, and six men lifted the king's bier and laid it in the wagon.

Now Atawulf laid his own shield at Alaric's feet—the old wolf's-head shield he had made when he first became a warrior. It was Alaric's now, perhaps to shield Alaric in that unknown realm of death, as Bold Wolf had often shielded him on the battlefield.

Others came forward with grave gifts to place in the wagon. Alaric's cupbearer, the half-Roman youth Aetius, brought his drinking cup of finely wrought silver to set beside him, and others brought silver plates and glass vessels, or carved figurines, or gold and silver coins. All went into the wagon.

At last, laden with its farewell gifts and precious burden, the wagon lurched into motion at Atawulf's signal, four strong mules straining to pull the iron-rimmed wheels over dusty, rocky terrain. An escort of two hundred horse warriors followed the line of two hills, and fifty captured Roman slaves on foot marched between, some carrying shovels slung over their shoulders, but most bare-handed and large-muscled. For this they were chosen—to dig the grave of the King of the Goths.

As the wagon rattled down the long draw, Winnifreya covered her shorn hair with the blue veil and turned blindly toward her tent. Singledia pressed a weathered, wiry arm around Winnifreya's shoulders, and the queen leaned upon her mother. Now her young daughters came to her side, she embraced them with one arm, and the four of them trudged together into the king's tent, Alaric's tent.

Dia's heart ached for them, and she discovered tears in her eyes, but she knew any comfort from her would be unwelcome and unneeded. She watched the wagon and Atawulf riding a black horse beside it until they disappeared over a rise in the hilly ravine.

• • •

Grimly Atawulf watched as the last flat slabs of rock were laid over the grave in the muddy riverbed. He never imagined such a dreadful task would be his, this covering with rocks the lonely tomb of his foster brother.

The river, shallow and sluggish after a dry autumn, had been easily dammed up and diverted by Roman slaves carrying and piling the great rocks. Now Atawulf was loath to give the order to dismantle the dam and allow the water to swallow the flat layer of rocks beneath which Alaric and his grave gifts lay buried.

A poor tomb for a King of the Goths, a mighty chieftain and warrior, a brother and friend, but Alaric must be buried, and on this the Goths were agreed: Romans must never find and desecrate the tomb of Alaric.

A distant murmur of thunder lifted Atawulf's gaze. To the east, above the higher mountain ranges, a blue-black veil of rain hung from massive cloud towers to sweep the jagged line of peaks. Rain in the mountains meant soon this wash would be a roaring flood as torrents raced down dry-packed ravines and riverbeds.

The time had come. Atawulf swept his arm toward the muddy bottom, and the slaves began heaving huge rocks off the crude dam and into the shallow depression they had dug. Soon the water trickled, then flowed, down the man-made ledge, swirling slowly over Alaric's rock-covered grave. One by one, the stones were plunked into knee-deep water, further obliterating the grave site, until the dam was destroyed and the stones lay scattered in the shallow water.

Atawulf stared at the ripples on the surface of the brown water; no trace of Alaric's grave or Alaric's life was written upon the river, and one good storm would wash away any trace of the work done here, of any tracks leading here.

Aye, no trace of the lively grin or step or handclasp, no trace of the robust laugh or shining awareness in those so brilliant eyes, no trace of him left at all.

Now the horse warriors marched the tired slaves away from

the river, far from the river, and if any slaves noticed that their trek headed not back toward camp but into a rocky gorge that gashed a jagged tear deep into the earth, they could but look at each other fearfully, for they had two hundred spears at their backs.

Atawulf glanced across the marching column to the other line of horses. Sigeric, teeth gleaming white in his ruddy face, grinned at him—a grin Atawulf had seen a hundred times before a raid on a villa or town.

Sigeric was going to enjoy this, and that fact Atawulf found disgusting. Yet on this they agreed: not one of these Roman slaves could live, carrying as they did the knowledge of Alaric's resting place.

Atawulf raised his good arm and the column halted. Sigeric watched him, eyes glittering under a fringe of red braids, challenge in his grin. Atawulf's gaze swept over the faces of the slaves, who were staring around in growing terror. Then he drew his sword and it keened death on the storm-laden air before he slashed out the throat of the nearest slave. The slaughter did not take long; horse warriors easily rode down fleeing men and dealt death with sword and spear wielded with cold fury and a thirst for vengeance.

As the warriors rode away from the remains of their butchery, Atawulf felt the first cold wind of the storm touch his back and heard thunder roll and crack like the wrath of God over his head.

9

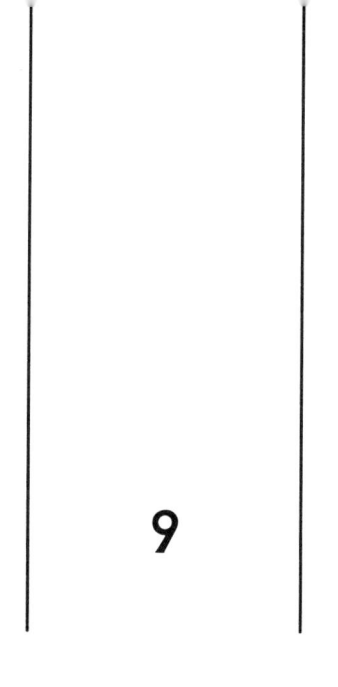

From her coach Dia saw the warriors return, Atawulf in the lead, and the wagon, empty now, clattering behind.

Grim and stern Atawulf looked beneath the black wolf's yellowed fangs and blood-red eyes, and behind him the blue-black sky flickered with lightning, as though beyond the jagged horizon giant blacksmiths forged and hammered iron.

Atawulf's face might well have been iron, and Dia felt his pain almost as if it were her own. The warriors were dismounting now, and she noticed bloodied spears and at least one horse with a blood-splotched coat. Before she could even ask herself what it meant, she knew. The Roman slaves were not with the warriors; they had not returned.

Forgetting her cloak, Dia burst from the coach and approached with determined steps. Weary of soul, Atawulf dismounted the black horse he rode.

Roman and Goth faced each other in the center of the camp.

"Where are the men you took with you?" Dia demanded. "The slaves?"

Atawulf regarded her darkly. His eyes were the same bruised color as the sky.

"Dead."

"You killed them?"

Atawulf's reply was stony silence.

"For God's sake, why?"

"They knew where Alaric is buried." He tried to brush past her, but she moved and stood before him.

"You murdered unarmed men to protect a *grave?*"

"Madam, we *butchered* them. We hacked them to pieces. Is that enough admission for you?"

"No, it is not enough! Innocent men are dead! How could you?"

"They were slaves, of no matter to Your Royalty."

"Slaves! They were human beings, and Romans! They were my people, and I was responsible for them!"

Atawulf stared at Dia as if she had sprouted a halo. "This is news to me. Aren't you the one who said a slave's life is worth less than a noble's?"

"I never said that."

"You as much as said it."

"*I* am not the one who cold-bloodedly killed fifty men for . . . for convenience!" Her voice lowered to an intense whisper. "How could I have ever thought . . . ?"

"Thought what?"

"That you were different! Less of a . . . savage!"

"Less savage? Than my own people? I'm a Goth, woman! I am what they are, and we are not interested in what Rome thinks. You easily forget, Miss Holy and Noble, that for centuries the Roman rabble has watched my people die in the arena for entertainment. That is not *savage?*"

"We . . . that is illegal now . . . we do not . . ."

"No," he snarled. "But as long as 'tis legal, eh? Like signing the death warrant of your own kinswoman? Was that not cold-blooded convenience?"

Dia struck at him then with her small fist, but his warrior's reflex was swift and he caught her slender arm in his right hand. His brawny hand held her fast no matter how she twisted to free her arm.

Movement made her turn her head. To her humiliation they had an audience. A large circle of warriors surrounded the two of them.

"Take your hand off me!" she gritted tightly.

"Never speak to me again of *savage,* Roman."

"You're hurting me!" she spat at him.

"Me? I'm just defending myself. If you twist your own arm, who's to blame?"

She glared up at him in fury, but she stopped struggling, her bosom rising and falling sharply with each angry breath. Even now Atawulf could feel desire for her, even in his hatred and his grief, and this thought fed his fury.

And Dia's eyes were held by the hot rage smoldering in those blue-black eyes, eyes mirroring the thunderclouds gathering around them. The air about them crackled with tension, light flickered at the edges of their vision, and she felt the leashed power within him, the strength and heat and motion.

Their gazes clashed, locked, and they stood glowering at each other in stubborn self-righteousness.

"Ve-ry sweet," a sarcastic drawl intruded. "I say lop off her head and send it to the Emperor as a token of our esteem."

Both startled gazes turned to face Sigeric, who sat forward in his saddle, leaning upon one knee. Dia shuddered; he reminded her of a hovering vulture, watching, waiting.

"*You* say? Since when, Sigeric?"

"Since we have no king."

Atawulf released Dia's arm and stepped away to face Sigeric squarely.

"I am your king."

"By whose authority?"

"Alaric's."

"Since when do the Goths let their chiefs be chosen for them? It has always been up to the warriors."

Atawulf looked around the circle of faces. He knew he could count on as many men here as Sigeric could—more, he would wager.

"True," he agreed, " 'tis the choice of the warriors." He swept his gaze from face to face as he spoke. "Alaric was thinking of that when he named me; he thought I was the man best able to lead you."

"Lead us where?" came a shout from one of the horsemen. A chorus of support echoed around the circle. "Tell us where!"

Dia had retreated until she reached Thalia and the coach. Now she climbed the steps and stood in the doorway on tiptoe, looking over the heads of the warriors at Atawulf in their center.

Atawulf stared at the ground a moment, then looked up at them again. "Where? I'd be lying if I said I knew where. But I can tell you, I hope to lead you to peace. Aye, a place to rest, a place to stop, an end to wandering and fighting for every last scrap. A place we can call ours."

Sigeric snickered. "What? Bold Wolf wants to be a farmer? A cattle herder?"

"So were our grandfathers, before the Huns rode over their lands."

"That's what peace got them. We are warriors; we take what we want."

"Because we have to. We have no place to stop and rest. We need homes and fields and cattle of our own. We'll have all the fighting we want defending them, I'll wager." He grinned at them. "How many of you would like to see your wives sweet-tempered and honey-tongued again? Or your children running and laughing in their own forests?"

The picture he conjured made them smile or murmur among themselves.

"First, we get out of Italia, where the Romans will be seeking us eventually. While the legions are tied up with invasions in Gaul, we'll seize our own piece of the Empire. But we must move quickly, for we don't know how long it might take Honorius to get up enough nerve to spare a legion or two against us. And right now, we've lost half our horses and too many men, and an attack now could finish us. Pray the Romans don't realize that till we're beyond the Alps."

He trod a circle, meeting their shining eyes. "I say we move, and move now, while we still can. Alaric entrusted me to take our people to safety, and on my oath that is what I will do! If any man objects, let him challenge!"

His words hung in the crackling silence, and thunder growled low on the horizon as Bold Wolf swept his storm-dark gaze around the circle and brought it to rest levelly on Sigeric.

"Do you challenge, Sigeric? If not, acknowledge me your king."

Sigeric's naturally ruddy complexion flushed deep crimson. He glowered at Atawulf standing before him so confidently. Then he nodded, eyes narrow and assessing.

"I challenge."

"I am in a mood black and foul today," Atawulf warned him. "If you challenge me now, will not be to first blood, Sigeric. 'Twill be to the death."

"To the death, then." Sigeric dismounted and drew his sword, and Atawulf reached across his body with his right hand to do the same. The pain in his left collarbone when he drew the heavy blade reminded him sharply of his bound and injured shoulder. No matter, he could best Sigeric one-handed, and with pleasure. He needed to hack at someone who could fight back.

The two warriors squared off, and Dia's breath caught in her throat. Then a scream of raw anguish ripped the air and froze the men in the clearing.

"*No-o-oo!*"

Winnifreya tore across the space and stood between them, hands outspread.

"*No!* Do not *dare!* Do not dare profane my husband's burial day! Alaric made his choice because he knew we must stand together, as one, so that we may all survive!" She spun and regaled Sigeric. "You are doing just what the Romans would wish us to do! Atawulf is right. We must be gone from here quickly. We need a leader, *now*, and Alaric chose Atawulf; if you choose to divide us now, Sigeric, you are destroying your people.

"And you," she said, whirling on her brother, "you, Atawulf, are just as bad. You're just prowling for a fight, hackles all up and teeth bared. I forbid it! I forbid it in the memory of Alaric, my husband, and I expect you to show more respect for my grief than this." Her voice caught, and she almost staggered under her loss, but she fought back the anguish. "I forbid it because I am your queen, and I will not stand by and see my people weakened and thrown into confusion while you two paw the ground and snort at each other like a couple of testy bulls!"

Winnifreya paused to take a breath and recover her temper, and from the outer fringes of the circle arose scattered and ragged feminine cheers and hand-clapping.

"I am Queen of the Goths, am I not?"

Voices rose in agreement, the deep drum of male voices blended with the women's. Winnifreya acknowledged them in one sweeping gesture.

"Then who will challenge me? Will you, Sigeric? Think of your people first, not your own glory. Put away your sword and save it for our enemies. Abide by Alaric's choice and save your challenge for another time, when we are safe out of reach of Rome, and," she told him pointedly, her voice trembling with barely controlled emotion, "when Atawulf is well recovered from his injury and the contest is more fairly matched."

"I can take him," growled Atawulf.

"You'll be dead next, Atawulf, and I can't stand it!" Winnifreya came near to weeping in her fury and her grief. She looked fragile and alone in the circle of warriors, her shorn hair shimmering around her head, but she looked magnificent to Dia. "You know you're sorely hurt, but you'd risk your life just to . . . just to show off!"

Atawulf turned around in surrender and buried the tip of his sword in the dirt. His sister never believed he could take care of himself, even now. It was easiest just to humor her. He rolled his eyes to low-lying heaven for sympathy.

Sigeric's face had darkened to a purplish hue, whether from shame or anger even he did not know, but he sheathed his sword and gripped the hilt hard. Truth, he had drawn sword on Atawulf knowing his opponent had but one free arm and a painful injury, and no, he would never have challenged Atawulf's sword otherwise. But clearly, the warriors would stand by Winnifreya, and her words pricked sharply at his pride. Glaring from Atawulf to his sister, he realized he must back down. Barely controlling his temper, he dipped his head curtly.

"Since you command me, my queen, I withdraw my challenge. Your authority I acknowledge."

"Then acknowledge Atawulf king. That also is my command."

Sigeric swallowed hard against the bitter words. "Aye, as you command me, I acknowledge Atawulf."

"*King,*" Winnifreya demanded to hear from his lips.

"Aye, king."

Atawulf nodded sharply and offered the man his hand. "Winn is right; this isn't the time for fighting. I need good captains, Sigeric. I'm counting on you and your men to cause such fear in the Romans that they will dread us more than the Devil himself. They must believe we are innumerable and everywhere; you're the man I need to accomplish that while we journey north."

"Aye," said Sigeric grimly, hearing at last words more to his liking. "Romans will tremble when they hear the name of the Goths, be sure."

Through bleak January the Gothic caravan moved north with all the speed thirty-odd thousand exhausted men, women, and children could make. They were weary and dispirited, virtually every one of them grieving for a drowned loved one, all of them mourning the death of their king.

Not a Goth did not know how vulnerable they were to attack, how great was the need to reach some safe haven soon. The highway thrust deep inland and then turned to run up the spine of the peninsula, slicing through the rugged southern ridges of the Apennines. They followed the paved road, for winter rains washed out lesser roads, and the highway led them through mountainsides once wild with oak and pine forests, but now cultivated with olive groves and vineyards.

The olive trees and grapevines offered but twisted branches barren and empty now, here in the midst of winter. The harvest was long gathered, and storehouses, scarce and far between, were half-empty.

Whether the Romans did indeed tremble at the approach of the Goths, they assuredly fled as news of their coming spread swifter than the long line of wagons and footsore vagabonds. And as the Roman people fled into the hills, they took as much of their winter stores as they could carry in their panic.

The homeless nation of Goths and straggling ex-slaves had by now devoured their own oxen—leaving wagons of possessions behind by the roadside, wagons of gold and silver and booty abandoned, useless—and now were reduced to roasting mule-flesh. Unthinkable to the horse warriors it was to eat the valiant war-horses, but winter grazing was scarcely enough to keep the steeds moving.

The Goths were close to starving, but the Romans must never know it, Atawulf thought grimly. That was one reason why he gave free rein to Sigeric in plundering the estates and villages. Atawulf in his turn led foraging parties for food, and his own frustration and desperation made even Atawulf a fell and heartquaking visage to the hapless peasants and village folk who ran afoul of his path.

The warriors torched the fields and villas, partly to scorch a path of destruction and terror about the caravan so that Rome or Ravenna might never learn the true weakened state of the Goths, but partly in sheer helpless anger at their inability to find enough food to stop the children crying at night and the women staring at them with fear-filled eyes and gaunt faces.

Worry gnawed at Atawulf; his people were weakened and dispirited. Speed, hunger, fatigue, and illness wore the Goths down. The highway became by turns a causeway which crossed wet, cold bogs, and a high ledge which hugged exposed, windbitten ridges. And now fever raged through the exhausted wanderers.

When he thought of their tragedies, of the broken ships and men, of Alaric dying believing he had failed his people, of their relentless journey to nowhere, Atawulf felt betrayed—betrayed by God, by Fate, by Rome.

And as ever when he thought of Rome, he thought of *her*. She had told him he was a fool if he believed she rejoiced in their losses. And now, in recalling her expression, he did believe her. But what could that matter? The hard fact was, she was Roman, and kin to that accursed Honorius, worst of the Imperials. And he hated Rome with every sinew and drop of blood in his body.

So why did he torture himself with her presence?

As a hostage she was useless—a hostage nobody wanted, not even her brother. Of course he would not kill her out of hand, as her brother deserved to have happen, but he found it difficult to explain to himself why he did not simply release her. But then she would be out of his reach forever. He wanted to know she was there, within sight, within reach, though he rarely acknowledged her, rarely spoke. He told himself he heeded Alaric's advice—someone, sometime would want her badly enough to bargain with the Goths. One day he would return her to Rome, to the Empire; why not do it now and release himself from this agony?

Impossible now, he argued with himself. She knew too much of their weaknesses to let her return to Rome now.

Meanwhile, the mere knowledge of her presence tormented him, for he was drawn to her like rain to Earth.

Dia felt like weeping over the scarred, scorched Earth. In the crimson sunset she could see the deliberate destruction of her country, her beloved Italia. And the suffering of her people was a sharp pain in her breast that never eased. The devastation of villas and villages, the burning of orchards and fields made her heartsick.

Priscus Attalus, who was native to this wild country, stared at the long line of fire on the black hills, a fierce streak glowing the same burning red as the sunset.

"Those are thousand-year-old oak forests. When I was a lad, all these valleys were oak forests, before they were cut for timber and left for pasture. They were thick with live oak and wildlife. I remember brown bear, wild stag, and deer, and forests awake with the chatter of raven and swallow. In those days we were wise not to travel alone, for fear of roving wolves taking solitary folk unaware.

"And now, even what's left of them is burning." The old man sighed, his thin shoulders drooping. "It will take years for the fields to recover—centuries for the forests."

Placidia glanced at Attalus beside her. The old statesman's love for the land and grief over its desolation creased his forehead and deepened the lines of his face. He did indeed love his country and his people, and his loyalty to them was beyond question. And to Attalus, Dia realized with new understanding, the land and the people *were* the Empire, and he felt no contradiction in defying even the Emperor, if it meant the protection of the Roman people. Thus he felt no treachery in accepting the title Emperor from the Goths, since Honorius had abandoned his people.

And it took courage to defy the Emperor and risk beheading for treason, his sure punishment if Honorius ever captured him.

"You are a faithful Roman, Priscus," she said suddenly. "I'm sorry I ever doubted your loyalty."

Priscus Attalus smiled warmly. "My dear Princess, you are forgiven. I knew from the start you shared my concern for the people. I hoped you'd understand."

"I understand a good many things now," Dia told him. She turned her gaze into the darkling night, black hills illuminated by blazing orange fires, their crests obscured by a choking curtain of smoke. "This enmity between Goths and Romans is destroying us—both peoples are suffering. And why? It seems so senseless."

Attalus shook his head sadly. He had no answer for her. Nor were there answers to the suffering she saw every day. And she knew Atawulf's grief; her heart ached for his pain. But why was he punishing *her?* He was being very unjust, and she was innocent of the terrible things he accused her of. Did he think no better of her than that?

But her eyes followed him whenever he came near. Grief seemed to weigh on his shoulders, burden his soul, and she wished she could ease his pain, but she had not that power. She could neither bring his brother back nor save his people, and these were the things that were bearing him down. And his people were worn and sick, Dia thought, and lost. She could scarcely complain of her crust of bread and cup of thin broth for supper. How many Goths went hungry this night?

• • •

She eyed Thalia's supper, not sure how much longer she dared sit and stare at it, but Thalia finally arrived, subdued and solemn. Dia had given her permission to visit Dulcie, and Thalia had found her friend shivering, sick and fevered, riding in an open wagon, huddled beneath a blanket.

Dia made Thalia take her to Dulcie, whereupon she bade Dulcie come ride in her coach, out of the weather.

Dulcie turned her head away. "No, miss, I can't."

"Can't? Nonsense, girl, of course you can."

"Won't, then, and 'tis unseemly of you to ask me."

"What? Since when is an act of kindness unseemly?"

"I'm a Goth now, miss," Dulcie said hoarsely. "I'm one of these." She nodded toward her companions in the wagon. "I want no special favors from you, begging your pardon."

Stunned, Dia reddened. Suddenly, she understood. Friendliness from the Roman Imperial embarrassed Dulcie among her own people. "Then I'll offer you no favors," she said stiffly, feeling ridiculously rejected. After all, it was absurd to feel hurt over a maidservant suddenly too good for her former mistress! She took her leave of Dulcie abruptly.

"Stubborn, foolish woman," she muttered, but she caught the anxious look in Thalia's dark eyes. "Perhaps if I send a blanket, she won't be too proud to take it from you, Thalia. Though I don't know why I bother, she's such an ungrateful wench. She won't thank me."

But Dulcie did accept the blanket from Thalia's hands, and she did send her thanks back to the princess. If Dia had been able to send food along, she would have, but the Imperial Princess shared the same dismal fare as the Gothic people; she had none but the inadequate handfuls doled out to her.

Thalia went to see Dulcie twice more, and the third time the handmaiden was gone overlong, well past the chilly nightfall. Dia sent Rayard to find her, and he returned carrying the slim, dark form in his arms, her straight black hair spilling over her face.

"She fainted," he told Dia gravely. "And her friend is dead—of the fever. Thalia stayed with her to the end."

"Poor dear," sighed Dia, thinking more of Thalia than of Dulcie. "Bring her in, Rayard, and I'll see she's warm, and there's barley broth for her. She's getting so thin, don't you think?"

Thalia awoke when Rayard sat her down in the coach, and she began to cry all over again. "She should have let you take her in, missy," she sobbed. "Why wouldn't she let you help her?" Thalia shook with ragged breaths. "She might be alive now, if she only . . ."

Grim, Rayard shook his head at the princess. "There's many of us dying of this fever, too many. Not much could've been done to help her, Your Royalty."

Dia nodded at him gratefully. "There, there, Thalia, did you hear Rayard? You did all you could for Dulcie. Here's your broth, now drink it down; it's not entirely cold yet."

Meekly Thalia drank the thin broth, then fell asleep under the blankets, but by early dawn she had thrown them off and was sweating all over. When Dia opened the window curtains to look at her, damp black hair plastered the hot flesh of her cheek and neck. Thalia complained that her head pounded horribly and her mouth was so dry she could hardly speak or swallow.

Dia brought her a cup of water and coaxed her to drink it all down, then Thalia fell back into fitful sleep. By the end of the day she was tossing and turning, burning and freezing by turns.

In desperation Placidia went to Singledia the Elder, who was herself busy with the contagion that vanquished the camp. Could she find Thalia a physician? Singledia shook her shorn grey head.

"We only have one physician who hasn't fallen ill, so we each do what we can. When her fever is high, cool her down with damp cloths. When she shivers with the chills, warm her with blankets. Give her water. Make her drink, and give her willow-bark tea. 'Tis all we have, but it's good for fevers, and 'twill help her head from hurting."

Dia took the offered bark and hurried back to her coach. She ordered Rayard to find her some charcoal, wood, anything to burn in the brazier, enough to warm the coach, and warm it all night. He built a fire outside, and soon collected enough smoldering wood and embers to fill the bronze brazier. Meanwhile Dia brewed a pot of willow bark over the campfire. Soon the coach was cozy and warm, and Dia had Rayard help sit Thalia up so she could give her the tea.

It hurt Thalia to hold her head up, and to swallow. Wishing she had some honey to ease the tea down, Dia coaxed her to drink. The night was long, Thalia restless and feverish, but Dia watched her and soothed her as Singledia had told her. Whenever Thalia struggled in her sweat-drenched blankets, Dia pulled them back and bathed her body with cool water, coaxing the heat out of her flesh, her too-thin limbs. And the moment Dia won one battle with the fever, a new one began, for Thalia would shudder and cry with chills while Dia fetched a dry blanket to wrap around her thin body. And Rayard sat vigil by the fire, keeping a bed of embers glowing sun-hot to fill the brazier throughout the night.

When day dawned, Thalia seemed no better. Her skin was still hot and damp to Dia's touch, even when she was shivering. Thalia cried, so wretchedly did her head hurt. She ached to the marrow of her bones, it seemed, and she could not hold her legs still. More willow-bark tea and wet cloths over her head helped ease her a little, then, suddenly, she was shivering and shaking with cold.

Dia wrapped another blanket around Thalia and bowed her head. In the night she had tried to pray, but her words were a distracted litany of terror. What if she should lose Thalia? She could not remember a time when the warm-hearted girl had not been right there beside her, sympathizing with her woes, sharing her joys, and now . . . now her handmaiden was her only real friend on this lonely journey. If Thalia died . . . oh, no, Dia could not bear thinking about the empty days and nights, the loss of that sweet smile, the silence of that gentle voice.

"Thalia, oh, my dear, sweet Thalia," murmured Dia, holding her sweat-damp hand, so hot and limp. "I'm sorry for ever slapping you, for every cross word I ever said to you. You're my dearest friend, and why do I only know it when I'm so close to losing you?" She stroked the fevered brow, smoothed the black strands back from the hot temple. "Please, don't leave me now. You don't want to die—I know it! What will I do . . . who will I laugh with or cry with . . . or . . . ?"

Unable to bear the thought, Dia fought back tears, sucked in a huge breath of determination.

"Thalia . . . Thalia, I forbid you to die! Do you hear me, I simply forbid it!"

Perhaps Thalia heard, for she turned in her sleep and moaned something hoarsely between cracked lips. Dia squeezed water from a cloth onto those fevered lips, but when Thalia tried to swallow, her throat convulsed against the raw pain and the liquid trickled from her mouth.

Now Dia gave in to her fear. Stumbling blindly, she flung open the door of the coach. Rayard leapt up from where he dozed by the fire, ready to shovel more coal into the brazier.

"Rayard, *please!* See if Singledia will come! I don't know what else to do!"

As Rayard dashed off, Dia sank to the coach steps wearily. "Mother in Heaven, please spare her," she prayed. "Thalia's so good; she's never hurt anyone in her life. Blessed Mary, I can't bear to see her suffering. I know I'm wretched and don't deserve her, but I beg you, don't take Thalia away from me. She's all I have."

Thus Atawulf found her, sitting desolate on the steps, head bowed, forehead pressed against hands locked in prayer. For several moments he simply rested his eyes on her, let the sight of her slender form touch his heart. She looked so fragile, her hair tumbling untended about her face and shoulders, her fingers clenched tight in desperation, so fragile he wanted to hold her in his arms and soothe her pain. And he knew what that pain was, for he had been there when Rayard came running for Singledia. His mother had shaken her head, wearied and overwhelmed by the countless folk she and Winn both tended. There was no more willow bark, no other medicine, and Singledia could do naught for Thalia that Dia was not doing already.

So Atawulf had come and found her sinking into despair. Eventually she sensed his presence and looked up with a start. Tears streaked her pale cheeks, glistened in her sea-deep eyes, and strands of dark-brown hair fell across the bridge of her nose. She pushed the wispy strands aside and gazed up at him hopefully.

"Is she coming?"

"She can't," he said gently. "You're doing all that can be done, she says."

"No, I'm not," Dia moaned. "I can't get her to drink anymore."

He held out his hand to her. "Let's see if I can."

She looked at him wearily, misery in her face. Sighing gratefully, she took his hand and let him pull her to her feet. They entered the coach, and Atawulf smoothed Thalia's hot brow. Carefully he lifted her into a sitting position, cradling her in one powerful arm.

Dia poured water from the pitcher and handed him the cup. Gently, persistently, he coaxed the water down her, and her swallowing appeared to become easier as the cool liquid slid down her throat.

Then he let her sink back onto the pillows and, as she was burning and sweating again, he took the wet cloth Dia passed to him and bathed her face and neck, shoulders and arms, to cool her down.

Dia watched him gratefully, for she had found it nearly impossible to lift Thalia's limp body and get her to drink. The water, at least, would give her weakened flesh something to fight the fever with. Dazedly, she saw Atawulf move toward her.

"You rest now," Atawulf told her. "You're worn out. I'll watch her."

He pressed her back toward her own bed. "Now you drink," he ordered as she sat down on the bed. He handed her the last of the water in a fresh goblet. "Have you eaten anything?"

Dia shook her head.

"I'll send someone to find you breakfast, if there is any. In the meantime, you sleep. You don't want to end up sick, too, do you?"

She shook her head again. Then she looked up at Atawulf tearfully.

"If she dies, I don't know what I'll do. I don't know how I'll bear it."

"I know." Oh, aye, he knew. He still felt the same about Alaric. He took her hands and lifted the cup, urging her to drink. Then he took the cup from her and swung her legs up on the bed. As she lay back on the pillows, he removed her slippers of soiled, worn satin, once a fine purple, now greyish and brown and worn through to the padding on the bottom.

She gazed up at him tiredly as his warrior's hands smoothed the hair from her brow. She felt better, now that he was here.

Her eyes misted and she sighed. She felt the strength in his broad hand clasping hers. She could trust Thalia to him for just a little while, just long enough to rest her eyes.

"You won't leave her?"

"No. I'll wake you if there's need."

She tried to nod, but her eyes closed and she was sinking through waves of light and shadow, lulling her worried mind into the peaceful dark.

Atawulf sat clasping her hand, watching her breathing deepen and slow, then he laid her small limp hand on the bed and pulled the coverlet over her sleeping form, careful not to disturb her rest.

Taking the pitcher, he hailed the nearest passing person to

refill it and bring something to eat, then he settled down on the floor of the coach, his hard-knit frame stretched across the open doorway because the coach was stuffy, and began his day-long vigil beside the sleeping princess and the feverish slave.

Thalia slept for now, and he left a cool damp cloth on her brow. Rayard returned; Atawulf ordered him to rest, but first he sent him with a message to Wallia. His brother must see that the camp was ready to move again tomorrow, whether folk were sick or not.

Atawulf knew he was pushing them. He was as tired and discouraged as they were. The voices of his people haunted him, asking constantly, pleading, *Where are we going? When will we stop?* He had no answers, no reassurances for them. He needed answers himself.

Atawulf fell into a brooding slump. His mind was exhausted, but he could not put the gnawing problems aside. His beard sank upon his chest and his eyes stared in unfocused reverie until the position pained his throbbing shoulder. Perhaps he had unbound it prematurely, but, dammit, he needed both hands. He shifted gingerly, suppressing a groan as he stretched and searched for a comfortable position.

He realized he had been staring a long time at Dia. His gaze lingered on her sleeping form, studying the way her rich brown hair spread out on the pillow. The soft curve of her cheek, the full lips parted slightly, like a sleeping child's. The dark fringe of lashes lightly touching the darkened flesh below her eyes, her face pale with fatigue, the furrow between her brows creased with worry.

He drank his fill of the sight of her while he could, like a thief at an unguarded well.

Thalia muttered and moaned, thrashing in her sleep, and Dia roused at the sound. She found Atawulf bending over her handmaiden, retrieving the fallen cloth. Dia forced herself to her feet and stumbled toward the bed.

Fever high, flesh hot and clammy, Thalia tossed her head from side to side, the bedding beneath her hair drenched. Dia took the cloth from Atawulf and wet it thoroughly in the water basin. Atawulf lifted the narrow shoulders in the curve of his arm and once more held her still and helped her drink the cool liquid. Water dribbled down Thalia's chin and she whimpered when she swallowed, but she drank thirstily. Then he watched as Dia moved the wet cloth over her handmaiden's hot flesh, and he was amazed at the gentleness of Dia's touch as she stroked the fevered woman and murmured soothing words, alternately urging her to rest and assuring her that she would soon feel better.

When Thalia rested once more, this time without succumbing to chills, Atawulf made Dia swallow dry barley bread and wash it down with weak wine. She insisted on staying awake to look after Thalia then. They sat in silence for a long while, Dia on the end of Thalia's bed, Atawulf on the edge of her own. Dia stared down at her laced fingers resting in her lap. What should she say? Atawulf's presence both confused and comforted her.

She looked sidelong at Atawulf in the afternoon light slanting through the windows. In the confines of the coach his warrior's strength seemed curiously transformed into a solid, steadying presence. The powerful energy within him easily flowed out in gentleness, and she marveled at the ease with which she leaned upon him.

"Thank you," she said at last.

He nodded gravely. "You've brought her this far."

Dia bit her lip and looked at Thalia's waxy face. "Are many people . . . dying?"

He hesitated, but decided on the truth. "Aye. But as many are pulling through."

"Oh, Thalia," she whispered, then self-consciously she turned to Atawulf. "I take so much for granted—I've done so all my life—but it seems a cruel lesson to only understand the important things just as they're slipping away."

"She's young and strong. Perhaps she isn't slipping away, Dia."

"If she isn't, I'll never take her for granted again. I can't remember a time when there was no Thalia, Thalia with her little sideways grin which always made me sure she was secretly laughing at me. I can't bear to think she could be gone . . . forever." Her last word ended on a little shuddering sigh, almost inaudible, but Atawulf heard it.

"Aye," he said thickly. Suddenly he leaned forward, elbows on knees, and reached out to take the hands she twisted in her lap. He held them in his broad palms, kneading her slender fingers gently. *You won't be alone,* he wanted to tell her. *I won't let you be alone.* But how could he promise her a thing like that, his enemy and his hostage? And what made him imagine that *he* could comfort her over the loss of someone who had a place in her heart?

Dia swallowed hard. Atawulf's kindness, this sudden tender touch, made her even more vulnerable to fear and sorrow. Tears welled in her eyes and threatened to overflow. She shook her head briskly and pulled her hands away, lest she break down altogether. Looking away, she dabbed at her eyes with the backs of her hands and then busied herself checking the temperature of Thalia's forehead.

This time, at Dia's cool touch on her brow, Thalia opened dark eyes, bright and lucid. She tried to move her thin dry lips, but Dia set a single finger to still them.

"Don't talk, Thalia. I'm here and I'm taking good care of you." When Dia squeezed water over the poor blood-cracked lips, Thalia managed a weak smile. Her hand fluttered up and rested against Dia's arm.

"There," said Dia chattily, trying to keep the tremor out of her voice as she pressed the wet cloth against Thalia's lips, "that's better, isn't it? You haven't been awake in so long, but now that you are, would you like a drink?"

To Dia's touch Thalia seemed not so hot as she had been, and when Atawulf sat her upright she drank thirstily from the cup Dia held. Then Dia fussed with the pillows behind her, and Atawulf eased her back into them.

"My poor Thalia," crooned Dia, smoothing the black strands back from her damp face. "You look exhausted. You need something to eat."

Mutely Thalia shook her head.

"Don't be ridiculous," Dia scolded. "Of course you do; you haven't eaten in two days, and how else will you gain the strength to . . . oh, Thalia, you are going to be all right, aren't you?"

Thalia's eyes slid closed; her head no longer hurt as if someone had piled a mountain on it, and the terrible ache had eased in her weak and listless limbs. She opened her dark eyes, jet black, all dilated pupil, and strove to focus on Dia's worried face. Thalia smiled her old smile, and in the pause Dia could still swear her maid laughed at her behind those shining eyes.

"Oat porridge, watered down," said a voice from the doorway. " 'Tis what we've been feeding the survivors." Singledia the Elder stepped into the coach.

"Survivors?" echoed Dia, finally realizing the import of Thalia's lucidity and the passing of the fever. The worst was over; Thalia was going to recover. The lump in her throat made her mute with emotion.

"Only half the sick are surviving. Your maid is one of the fortunate ones."

Atawulf gruffly voiced what his mother left unspoken. "She had good care."

Dia blinked rapidly. Silly to cry, she thought, when the danger was past. Busying herself with the water pitcher and cloth, she furtively dabbed her eyes with a damp corner of the material, but Thalia did not miss the gesture. When Dia brought the cloth near her forehead, Thalia reached up and caught her hand, pressed it against her warm cheek.

"Miss Dia," murmured Thalia, "you were here all the time . . ."

"Well, of course I was," Dia replied saucily. "And you must admit, I'm an excellent nurse, am I not?" The princess was beaming.

"Oh, miss, thank you ever so . . ."

"Thalia, don't be maudlin. You know very well I had no intention of letting you die and leave me here all alone. Besides," Dia said, glancing at the man who filled her awareness with his presence even as she had slept, "you should thank Atawulf as well. He's been here all day."

Gratefully Thalia thanked the king, though she knew well for whose sake he had kept his vigil.

Now Singledia the Elder turned to her son. "Atawulf, our people cannot go on. This order to move on tomorrow is going to break them. They wonder where you are taking them and to what purpose."

Atawulf's sigh was soul-deep. "Mother, I wish I knew. I only know we can't stay here. We're too close to Rome, too near the highways. Troops could come out of Ravenna anytime to cut us off; our only chance is to cross the Tiber and go north into Umbria, where the drought did not hit so hard."

" 'Tis too late for that," Singledia told him gravely. "We will all die before Umbria."

Bold Wolf simply sat and stared at her for a moment, then, propping his elbows on his knees, he dropped his head into his hands, rubbing his eyes with the heels of his palms. Dia had never seen him look so defeated, his brawny shoulders hunched as though Atlas himself had never carried a greater burden.

He raised his head; his blue eyes stared out the open doorway.

His mother's throaty voice gently but persistently prodded him. "Can we stop here and dig in? Let the healthy construct ditch, scarp, and rampart, and let the weak and the sick rest."

Atawulf's lips drew back, a smile of grim irony. "We have defeated ourselves. We raided this area during the siege of Rome and put the fields to the torch. Now we reap what we've sown. There's not enough food in a hundred miles to sustain us. Mother, I've searched for some place we can hold, some place we can recover from our wounds, but not here, not out in the open like this!"

His voice was a groan of pain. "We must move tomorrow and look for some safe place. We have no choice. A place we can defend, walls we can defend, high ground if we can find it, with shelter from rain and wind and spying eyes, stables for the horses—who are stumbling on their last legs and far from battle-ready—someplace with a good store of grain . . ." His voice trailed off; he shook his head wearily. "If such a place exists."

Silence hung in the coach like cold shadows. Atawulf felt cold, but he clenched fist and jaw and girded his spirit to go out and face his people. Then a voice, soft and sure, dispelled the shadows.

"I know of such a place."

Atawulf turned, startled, to face Galla Placidia. Seated at Thalia's bedside, hands clasped in her lap, the Imperial Princess of Rome regarded him with clear, grave eyes.

"What?"

"I know of such a place," she repeated steadily.

"Where?"

"First you must swear to me that your men will harm none of the occupants, will destroy nothing, burn nothing—if they have not already."

"You're sure about this place?"

"Yes. I . . . I know it as well as I know my own . . ." She had been about to say "heart," but did she know her heart anymore? Was this a traitor's heart?

But it came down to this: he had come to her aid; now she would come to his.

"Where is this place?"

"First, your word, King of the Goths."

"Aye, my word on it; we will destroy nothing, harm no one." Then he hesitated. "*If* we meet no resistance."

She shook her head. "You will meet no resistance."

"Then you have my word."

She nodded. "It is north of here."

Singledia asked the question most urgent to her. "How far? We cannot travel much further."

"If we are as near to Rome as I think, then two or three days."

Atawulf frowned. "Two or three days north will bring us to Rome itself."

"Nearly. We will make for Tivoli."

He looked at her doubtfully. "Woman, we could be trapped between Rome and Ravenna."

"I know a place. You have *my* word, Atawulf."

His dark blue gaze, beneath hawk-winged brows, penetrated hers. Slowly, he nodded.

"I will bring a map," he said. "Show me the best route."

And their eyes held a long moment before breaking the sudden link between them, Atawulf full of the knowledge that she trusted him on his word alone, Dia full of the knowledge that he would place his people's fate in her hands, on her word alone.

And as her gaze dropped to Thalia's solemnly approving stare, Dia fervently prayed that she was right, that this haven still stood undiscovered and undisturbed, and that it was indeed safe from attack by the legions.

10

The Gothic caravan slogged up gentle slopes of rain-soaked grass, winter-brown pastures flattened and dead, on a cold, blustery day. An ocean of grey clouds scudded high over an enormous wall which stretched in unbroken smoothness in either direction.

Atawulf, sitting on horseback on the slope below the structure and bending his neck back sharply to study the straight plane of the stones, estimated that wall to be five times the height of a Gothic warrior.

His hopes rose considerably. Perhaps this villa would be as suitable and defendable as Dia said it would. He prayed it was also as well-stocked as she claimed.

At his side, Wallia let loose a long, low whistle of admiration. "Her Royalty sure knows her villas."

Atawulf glanced at his brother. "We haven't seen the rest of it yet."

Wallia grinned. "Want to wager on the rest? I'm ready to bet 'tis as good as this—or better."

Atawulf shook his head. "That would be one bet I'd hope to lose." He turned and gazed back down the long, easy slope that was the base of the hill. The caravan—wagons, horses, and staggering folk half-dead on their feet—formed a wide, straggling arc as it turned west along the rolling foothills. The nearest entrance to the villa proper was there, where Dia had directed them, up the hill.

"Come on," Atawulf said with a jerk of his head. "We don't want Her Royalty taking charge of the whole caravan at the gate."

The brothers rode along the wall until they reached a sharp right angle. Then the whole western wall of the villa filled their vision. At the far-distant end an imposing structure jutted out at double height, and the upper part appeared to be nothing but window after window overlooking the lower slopes.

Now it was Atawulf's turn to whistle. "Is this a villa or a *fortress?*"

In the wide open pasture before the villa—an area of twenty acres at least—the Gothic nation was gathering, the thickest snarl of humanity crowding around a large irregular-shaped building jutting out from the wall.

Atawulf touched his heels to the sides of the black and picked his way through knots of exhausted people who huddled on the ground where they stopped, pulling cloaks around them against the chill wind whistling across the open space. He and Wallia wove a path through the disorganized tangle of mounted warriors, wagons, men and women to the building where one man at the gate held back the tide of Goths like a rock catching logs and damming a river.

"I'm sorry, nobilissima," the man said, swallowing convulsively and eyeing the barbarian flood converging around him. "I am not allowed to open the gates to an army of Goths, only to the Imperial family. Your Sacred Person may enter, but not... not..."

The man stared past the Imperial Princess and his face paled nearly as white as his eyes. Who was this hawk-browed, grim-visaged warrior for whom the others parted?

Atawulf studied him impassively from horseback. The guard wore the white plume of the Protectors, though he seemed well past the age when he should have retired and returned to his ancestral estates.

"Don't be ridiculous," Placidia argued. "Your handful of men cannot possibly hold off an army of seasoned warriors, and King Atawulf has given me his word that if you open the gates peacefully no one will be harmed."

The warrior on the black horse bared his teeth, and the terrified guardsman was certain this was the dreaded barbarian king.

"Nobilissima, please," the guard whispered. "My duty . . ."

"Is to obey the Imperial Princess," Dia snapped more sharply than she intended. She was cold to the bone standing here wrapped in her warmest green woolen cloak, and her head hurt, a dull ache she had tried to ignore all afternoon. All she wished was a place to lie down and some hot honeyed wine to soothe the rawness in her throat. Dia sighed and beneath her cloak clasped her fingers tightly together to keep from shaking with cold.

"I promised the king there would be no resistance," she said with all the patience at her command.

"You call this resistance?" drawled the king's voice from behind and above her. He peered through the narrow entrance into the courtyard where a handful of guards waited, gripping javelins. He could see their knees knocking from here.

She did not turn to look at Atawulf; her head hurt when she turned too abruptly. "Captain," she addressed the frightened guardsman in that tone of hers which conveyed that every drop of blood in her veins was twice royal and he would best heed it, "do you wish to die needlessly when you have only to obey an Imperial command?" The white plume shuddered in negation. "Very well, I, Galla Placidia, *command* you to stand aside and let us enter."

With visible relief the white plume waved wildly, then

dipped and very nearly brushed the flagstone as the captain bowed and stepped shakily aside. The remaining Protectors hurriedly parted to either side and leaned on their javelins as though their knees had at last failed them. No man wanted to be spitted on a Goth's sword to defend an untenanted villa.

They were too old for useless heroics, thought Atawulf as he dismounted and led his horse through the rounded archway. And if he thought every one of them had spent his entire twenty-five-year career guarding a mostly empty villa, he was right. None of them had seen any more action than the annual summer procession of Imperial princesses.

Placidia proceeded with slow steps, fighting a wave of weakness behind a mask of determined dignity. She led the way into the large open courtyard adjacent to a large hall.

Dia made for that roofed hall wearily, head pounding, cursing her weak body for succumbing to fever. She *hated* this miserable feeling, this mind-numbing weight in her head, and her inability to shake it off.

Within the shelter of the hall she found she could go no farther and sank onto a marble bench as though her body collapsed there of its own volition. She wanted just to sit a moment, she told herself, and steady the spinning sensation in her head.

Atawulf laid a broad hand upon her forehead, causing a gasp of shock from the guardsman.

"Do you have medicines here?" the king demanded of the captain. "And a physician?"

Before the captain could answer, a stately old man was crossing the hall toward them as fast as his ancient bones would allow.

"Yes, yes," the man spoke as he approached, having taken in the situation. He bowed swiftly, but slightly, bending only so far as a man of his age need concede. "We have medical supplies and the servants' physician. Mistress Placidia, I'll send for a litter immediately to carry you up the hill."

Dia looked up at the old man and managed a smile. "I had no

idea you kept a litter here, Sylvanus. Isn't that a sort of sacrilege?"

"We have one, nobilissima, though I daresay it hasn't been used over twice in a hundred years. A very pregnant noblewoman, I believe, required . . ."

"Old man," a growl of impatience interrupted him. "Your princess is in need of rest. Stop jabbering like a jaybird and see to it."

The elderly man drew upon decades of dignity and eyed the barbarian with an affronted glare, then he glanced quizzically at the Imperial Princess.

"Sylvanus," Dia told him, "this is His Majesty Atawulf, King of the Goths. He and his people are my *guests*." She cut her eyes warningly at Atawulf. "Sylvanus has been steward of this villa since my grandmother Justina's time."

"*Before,* if you please, nobilissima," the old steward corrected her.

"This is his domain. No one disputes him here except—"

"Ah, Mistress Placidia!" exclaimed a breathless, quavering voice as an ancient bag of a woman bustled between the men. "A miracle, it is, to see you again!" The woman was all loose folds of skin and sagging wrinkles—and wreathes of smiles. She scurried forward and wrapped large arms around the seated princess. So short she scarcely bent at the waist, she seemed all bosom.

Dia accepted this smothering embrace with an unexpected relief and suppressed tears.

"Chrysanthia," the princess murmured, her voice muffled against the ample shoulder.

"Why, my dear, you're trembling—and hot!"

"Actually, I feel quite cold . . ."

"You're burning up with fever." The grey-haired woman turned a wrathful glare upon the old steward. "Don't you realize this child is ill? Send for the litter!"

"I just have," Sylvanus answered quickly. "It'll be along any moment."

Now the brown-eyed wrath turned upon Atawulf. "Have you been dragging this child about in this weather knowing how sick she is? What kind of treatment is that for an Imperial Princess of Rome? Are you barbarians that heartless and cruel . . . ?"

"Chrysanthia," Dia half-laughed, half-scolded, "I've only just become ill, and this person you are accosting as though he were a ruffian is the King of the Goths."

The squat little crone faced him squarely. "Begging your pardon, but barbarian *kings* have no right to be carrying off *Imperial Princesses* in the first place. He didn't do anything ungentlemanly to you, did he, honey?"

Dia shook her head, then regretted the movement. "No, no, King Atawulf has been the impeccable *gentleman*," she said, knowing how that would gall him. "Please treat him as an honored guest—and his people. Many of them are ill and in need of warm rooms."

Chrysanthia looked beyond the king and surveyed the hall filling up with barbarians—men, women, and children—all looking ragged, cold, and half-starved.

"Sylvanus," she snapped up at the old steward, "don't just stand there. Find these people places to sleep." She turned her attention to a slave who had come in on her heels. "Fidus, see the fires are stoked and inform the cooks we've guests to feed." At last she stared up into the face of the king. "How many folk are you, anyway?"

"About thirty thousand," Atawulf answered gravely.

"Good Lord!"

"Nobilissima," quavered the old steward unhappily. "We have stores, but not that many. Our funds from the Sacred Largess have been shortened these last few years . . ."

Dia closed her eyes and leaned her head back against the hard, cold marble of the wall behind the bench. "Please, Sylvanus, take it up with King Atawulf. I'm just . . . tired."

"Of course you are," fussed Chrysanthia, glaring at her husband. "We've plenty for a few days at least, if they don't mind stretching a meal or two with boiled wheat."

Atawulf almost admitted boiled wheat was worth its weight in gold to the hungry Goths, but he caught himself and merely nodded. "It'll do."

Sylvanus nodded, his turn to chide his wife. "Chrysanthia, you ninny, the Goths are warriors. They *prefer* good army fare, not fancy dishes all done up. Am I right, Your . . . Your Majesty?"

"You are right," grinned Atawulf, deciding he liked the old steward.

The voices around Dia threatened to dissolve into a meaningless buzzing. "My coach is outside, Chrysanthia. Have someone fetch Thalia so she can go up in the litter with me. She's been ill and I wouldn't let her leave the coach."

"Oh, is that dear girl with you, miss? Don't you worry, I'll see to it immediately."

Dia sighed and leaned listlessly against the cold wall, letting the sounds of chaos clutter the air about her heavy, pounding head. She fought the urgent longing just to lie down on the hard bench and give herself up to shivering misery, but she would not.

At last the litter arrived; Atawulf and the steward's wife helped her step into the musty old conveyance, its ornate gilded posts and rich tapestries coated in years of dust. As she crumpled upon the sea of pillows she dimly heard the steward prattle on about it dating back to Queen Zenobia's time, and she laughed to herself at the notion that she shared both Zenobia's cushions and Zenobia's dust.

"What's she laughing at?"

"Hush, you old fool, the poor child's half out of her head with fever."

The last clear thing in Dia's awareness was Thalia's arrival and her maid's deft hands supporting the ringing, pulsating, torturing thing that was her head as it lolled off the pillows. The uneven lurch and sway of the litter was sickening, and her stomach felt violated.

The trip was interminable, and long before the hastily gathered litter-bearers had wound between the buildings and gardens of the villa, long before they set the heavy litter on the richly inlaid floor of the sumptuous Imperial apartments, Dia had vomited on the silken pillows and cried bitterly against the hateful helplessness and unrelenting misery.

Atawulf watched Dia being carried away in the litter, followed by the astonishing ball of energy that was the steward's elderly wife. The Imperial Princess was in good hands, the best, he felt sure, especially with Thalia at her side. It was time to turn his full attention to the sheltering of his people.

They trickled into the hall, staggering with weariness, lugging only the most necessary possessions, and the trickle spread slowly and steadily from the hall, filling the vast, intricate maze of buildings and plazas, gardens and colonnades as completely and thoroughly as rising floodwaters.

And what a maze it was! Like no other villa Atawulf had ever seen, and had not old Sylvanus been guiding him and discussing the purpose and suitability of each building as they passed, he would have been lost in this huge complex.

This was neither villa nor fortress, Atawulf decided, but a *city*, a city designed for luxury. Fortunately the steward was there to lead them toward the most useful of the buildings—libraries, theaters, reception halls, baths, dining rooms—anything that would provide a roof and walls for the multitudes of Goths.

And the weary multitudes seemed scarcely to notice the exquisite fountains and pools, graceful statues and columns, shaded arcades and gardens, which were set like gems between the buildings. Around each corner they stumbled, into each new structure, where they dropped upon tastefully marbled floors beneath elegantly carved roofs supported by gold-trimmed columns. They spread their blankets, opened their sacks of hard bread, hung wet clothes over gilded balconies and stairs, rocked their children, dipped clear water from fountains splashing over fanciful statuary, tended their sick, mourned their dead, and hoped they would not be required to move on again too soon.

Warriors watered their horses in huge clear pools artfully ringed in columns, set the animals free to wander on sloping lawns and in gardens crisscrossed with paved walkways.

By the time Sylvanus led Atawulf through the Imperial apartments, the King of the Goths had long since stuffed his amazement into a corner of his mind and concentrated on the usefulness of the innumerable rooms. They passed through no less than four huge peristyles terraced upon the higher slope, each private garden enclosed by its own quadrangle of richly decorated apartments. The Imperial apartments were grouped around the farthest and most magnificent garden. Here, Sylvanus told him, the Imperial Princess would be put to bed in the "Emperor's Rooms." By now Atawulf had no need to ask which Emperor the steward referred to, for the walking encyclopedia of villa lore had scarcely spoken of any Emperor but Hadrian.

Dusk was rapidly darkening the sky by the time Atawulf, with his mother and sister, began an organized effort to move the weakest and most ill of his people into the four vast complexes of rooms which formed the luxurious guest quarters of the villa. Here, in richly decorated accommodations, the sick were laid in gold-footed beds. Here, too, intricately patterned floors were warmed from below as slaves stoked and fanned the fires, heating musty, disused air ducts beneath the expensive mosaics.

The scouting parties Atawulf had sent galloping out when they first spied the walls returned in half-light. They had circled the outside perimeter of the villa, found it secure, and posted guards as ordered.

As darkness settled over the hills, slaves seemingly appeared like magic out of shadowy corners and set the buildings aglow with torches and oil lamps. With an almost audible relief the Goths broke out their meager suppers, added to by silently gliding slaves carrying bowls of dried fruit and pickled eggs and onions. At last Atawulf found a moment to breathe easily and decide that they were as secure as they could make themselves this night; before sinking into sleep upon a handy dining couch he charged himself to awaken in a few hours for the change of the watch. The clouded sky darkened from indigo to black, and if any one of the Roman peasant folk had remained on the plain below after the passing of the Goths, he would have been amazed to look up and see the villa alight as it had not been since Hadrian's day.

In the days that followed, Atawulf and his people explored every square foot of the rambling jumble of architecture and nature that was Hadrian's Villa.

One hundred and fifty acres, Sylvanus informed him amid a deluge of details on his world. Seven square miles of gardens and walkways, covered arcades and riding parks, pools and waterfalls, tiny temples nestled in hidden grottoes. Vast expanses of patterned pavement floored great open plazas, plazas bordered by long arcades and balconies. Incredible structure after structure met Atawulf at every turn, each one as beautiful as the last, each one seemingly designed to draw the eye along pleasing views to the next.

Theaters and libraries, baths and dining halls formed miniature forums of their own. Adjoining the largest bath complex Atawulf discovered a huge swimming pool in its own tree-shaded park, surrounded by two floors of colonnaded arcades. Nearby he came upon a round open-roofed pavilion encircled by a moat of crystalline water. As the tiny island pavilion seemed more open space and columns than shelter, and was tucked away out of the regular flow of foot traffic, the Goths had little use for it and left it vacant.

At the opposite end of the villa, Atawulf and Wallia found a great oblong pool nestled in a narrow valley. The placid surface of the water reflected in pristine detail exquisitely carved statues standing around the pool's perimeter, each statue framed by a shapely arch supported upon elegant columns. On a flat rock in the middle of this fanciful pool, a great crocodile raised its head to the sun.

Atawulf and Wallia glanced at each other in simultaneous challenge. Grinning, they plunged into the pool, splashing silver spray over the marble statues, and swam like mad for the rock. Wallia reached the rock a length ahead of Atawulf, whose left arm was still stiff from injury. The brothers laughed as they pulled themselves onto the rock, where the life-sized crocodile sculpted entirely of green marble basked in late-winter sunshine.

Wallia pretended to wrestle the beast and placed a dripping, booted foot upon its marble head in victory, but Atawulf goosed him and dumped him back into the cold water. Atawulf laughed hugely at his sputtering brother, and his brother joined his laughter, their matching blue eyes meeting in merriment. Then, as abruptly as it started, their laughter died, they sobered, each thinking the same thing.

Alaric would have loved this! He would have won the race, too.

Suddenly Atawulf bared his teeth at his younger brother and challenged, "Race you to the *end!*" On the last word he dived off the rock and sliced into the water. With a yell Wallia plunged in after him, but Atawulf pulled himself up onto the far rim before his brother could even touch it.

"Cheat!"

"Slugbrain!"

"Old man!"

"Aye, and wily, don't forget." Atawulf looked over Wallia's shoulder at a structure built into a low hill. "Turn around; just look at this thing!"

They stood before a man-made cave hollowed into a small hill. The room-sized cavern was honeycombed with channels through which waterfalls bubbled and tumbled and pooled and spilled around the sides, and splashed down on either side of a floor built in the lee of the circular cave; in the midst of this cavern of rippling water were stone couches set in a semicircle.

"What's this?" wondered Atawulf, his words nearly lost beneath the play of waterfalls.

"Looks like a dining room."

Atawulf grimaced, dripping and shivering in the open air. "Cold eating—water everywhere." Now Atawulf gazed about him, stopping to stare into glittering sunlight glancing off the long pool. Aye, water everywhere. Come to think of it, the whole damn villa was running all over with water.

Pools, moats, fountains, channels—the sound of water was everywhere, filling the air with water-song, soothing the soul, whispering of peace and rest. And healing. And the Goths, surrounded by that constant lullaby, were healing.

The place must be magic, Atawulf thought. Or a gift from God. It was the miracle his people needed. It was sanctuary.

"How did we miss this place on our forages?" he mused to Wallia.

"Hard to imagine, but it *is* off the highways and partly hidden by these hills. Lucky we found it."

"No, we're lucky Dia—Her Royalty, *led* us to it."

"Aye, I almost forgot. I guess I win that bet."

"What bet?"

"That 'twould be even better on the inside."

"You're right. She knows her villas. And she'd say, 'I told you so,' if she could—if she knew." Atawulf's face folded into deep creases; he suddenly looked his age.

"Mother says she'll pull through, Bold Wolf. Ma ought to know."

Atawulf nodded. "Aye, I know, but I won't feel easy till her fever breaks."

Atawulf was keenly aware that Dia loved this place and its people, and that she had opened her home to him, to all the Goths.

Strangely affected, he felt she had given him a great treasure, one dear to her heart, and she had shown him a depth of trust he had never expected. *God, let her live. Give me a chance to . . . To what?*

"You all right?" Wallia studied him with concern.

"Aye, aye. She . . . she did right by us."

Wallia nodded, saying nothing, but briefly clasped his older brother's shoulder. Wallia understood him more than he knew.

Atawulf turned wearied eyes toward him, deep blue wells of great heart, of grief, worry, and resolve. "I worry too much, brother. I'm not God, just a warrior. Best stick with matters warriors understand. Come on, let's find out where all this water comes from."

This magnificent villa to which Dia had led them sprawled on the gentle southern slope of the foothills, so that it lay on high ground, but at the same time its varied terrain was cradled in a natural bowl scooped between rises. Two streams hugged the shallow valley and, with the help of a graceful aqueduct, fed the villa's many waterways.

Beyond the rambling enclosure formed by walls, buildings, and colonnades, they discovered more of the grounds—ornamental gardens laid out in geometric precision, tree-lined avenues for riding out into the countryside, orchards of bare-branched fruit trees standing row upon row, crowded kitchen gardens, too, with soil already fresh-turned for early planting.

The Goths found winter stores within the walls, jar upon jar of staples in a hundred and more rooms underground, dark, cool rooms where stores of pickled eggs and vegetables, honeyed fruits and cheeses were stacked near to the ceilings. Here they uncovered a larder to feast an Emperor and his companions—and all his horse, too. They found granaries stocked with barley, oat, and wheat.

Grain to feed their hungry children, grain for bread, grain for stew, grain to feed their thin war-horses.

The villa contained stables for two hundred horses, and Atawulf made good use too of the buildings and arcades. Colonnades around courtyards and gardens he used to shelter the animals from a smattering of wind and rain, but with the arrival of spring, the sky seemed to have given up drenching the land and instead bathed it in sunlight. Everywhere in the villa were sunlit gardens, pools and fountains, and everywhere they put the horses.

Atawulf filled the four grand peristyles with horses, which pleased the many families crowded into the royal quarters, whose rooms all opened into the gardens, for they were accustomed to living with their horses and not inclined to do without them now.

Horses sunned in a huge formal garden laid out like a mosaic. They rolled and stretched in the long riding park shaped like a stadium racecourse. They trotted across the lawn of the spacious park surrounding the Emperor's private swimming pool, overlooked by double-tiered colonnades for the Emperor's private promenades.

The Emperor's private bath and the great bath complex Atawulf had reserved for the people, for these were two more buildings in which the floors could be heated, and the old and the ill needed the warmth.

The villa seemed to work a sort of magic on them beyond the sheltering roofs, warm rooms, and plentiful food. The lulling peace of whispering waters, the trees and lawns, the quiet hillside—the villa seemed permeated with a peace so deep that they breathed it in the air, drank it in the waters, until peace seeped into their heavy hearts and melted the burdens they had carried for so long.

Aye, the people were healing. He found that heartened him, knowing they grew stronger daily. It gave him new hope, and new resolve. He bent all his energy now toward the preservation of his people. After a few days of rest for everyone, he sent out patrols. The Goths had to supplement the villa's stores or they would be too quickly emptied, therefore Atawulf himself rode out to demand tribute of Tivoli and other nearby towns.

Wisely the towns paid up. Rome, however, was more obstinate. The city closed silent gates against them, the walls stood faceless and voiceless. Atawulf took this with good humor, suspecting that the Senate was in frantic argument and would be for a good year, so he passed up Rome and relieved Ostia of its grain stores.

They raided the countryside—villages, estates, farms. Atawulf divided the horse warriors into foraging parties, sending them raiding far afield, striking at lightning speed; to the Romans he wanted it to seem as if the Goths were everywhere, everywhere at once, too many to count, too fierce to resist.

He gave Sigeric charge of the raiding parties, for this was what he and his men were best at. Atawulf hated to admit it, but he needed the kind of horror Sigeric could stir in the hearts of the people. They would not forget Sigeric, though Atawulf constrained his captain to kill only when resisted, only if it could not be avoided. He wanted fear, not disgust. Fear enough to make the Emperor hesitate, not so much disgust that he would feel pressured to send legions after them.

Atawulf reminded the warriors of that when he sent several bands raiding north into rich and fertile Umbria. He gathered them in the grand plaza, as he thought of it, high on the slope. It was a great square enclosed by the usual colonnade, but at one end rose the most enormous, fantastic building. Its center was a vast dome spanning a daunting distance, seemingly held aloft by nothing more substantial than a few sweeping rows of slim columns. So light and delicate did they appear that Atawulf looked up again and again to ascertain that the pillars were not merely decorative, but supporting the entire dome in an elaborate architectural feat, a design both incredibly strong and beautiful.

Atawulf whistled, deliberately, a hawk's whistle, for this was the dome that sang, and his whistle reverberated shrilly, ringing the dome like a great bell. He howled, a wolf's howl, and the dome howled, like echoes in a deep cavern. He shouted.

"I am Atawulf!"

And the dome rang with the voices of ghosts, haunting, *wulf, wulf, wulf* . . .

Atawulf gazed up at the domed ceiling, wondering. Here Atawulf most felt the ghost of Hadrian. The soul of a man who built such magnificent things simply because he wanted them to be. A man who stood on these very tiles, looked up into this very dome, which he had conceived and conjured for his pleasure.

Atawulf knew he, himself, could never have created this dome, nor its many adjoining rooms seemingly designed to do no more than play with sunlight, nor the buildings on the slope below it, nor anything—not one thing—in this fantastic villa.

And the thought saddened him. He heard Dia's voice, scathing: "Romans build civilization, you Goths only destroy it." And he knew she was partly right.

What would Hadrian, Emperor of Rome, think of Atawulf, King of the Goths, standing boldly beneath his dome, reviewing Gothic cavalry in his grand plaza?

"Swear to me you won't destroy it," Dia had said.

And he understood. Atawulf, King of the Goths, could not build beauty out of stone, but he could see the beauty. The order and the purpose of each structure almost disguised by the sensuous play of curve and line. Aye, he understood. He could not create it, but he would never destroy it.

For a passing moment he envied Hadrian his creation, his world, his Empire, but he shook it off. He was Bold Wolf, King, and Hadrian was three centuries dead, and Rome couldn't even evict a few thousand hungry Goths from the Emperor's magnificent villa.

Atawulf laughed. He hoped the ghost of Hadrian heard him. *I have your villa, Hadrian! Come take it back!*

The great bell rang with his laughter. And Atawulf felt a sudden kinship to Hadrian the Emperor, who came out to this very courtyard and addressed his personal troops, just as Atawulf rallied his warriors. A fighting man, he recalled, leading the legions of Rome in her glory.

Glory, hell. Conquerors, hell. Bloody band of Roman

thieves, like the brigands Dia accused the Goths of being, only more of them, bigger raiding parties.

A King of the Goths had every right to stand tall before an Emperor of Rome.

He turned to go, to speak with the men on horseback milling and buzzing in the plaza, but then his glance fell upon a young trumpeter holding the great horn of the Goths, and he motioned the youth into the center of the domed hall.

"Blow the cavalry charge. Blow it so that even Hadrian knows we are here."

Proudly, nervously, the young trumpeter raised the heavy horn to the high dome and blasted the air with the dreadful bellow of the Gothic charge.

Beware! Beware! The Goths are upon you!

And the great dome took the sound and amplified it and shook the stones of the courtyard with it, and the trumpeter grinned at his king, and in the plaza horses' ears pricked and hooves stamped, and every man's talking ceased, and every man's eye turned toward the dome.

And in this mood, when he emerged full into the grand courtyard packed with war-horses and warriors bedecked in a wild array of armor and color—in this mood Atawulf sent them forth toward Umbria with a bellowing command:

"Show Rome that the Goths do not fear her, do not love her, will never serve her!"

And in this mood still, after the excited warriors galloped out from the villa with whoops and shouts, after Priscus Attalus met him striding along the crooked pathway which wended the narrow parkland called the Vale of Time, after he slowed and strolled with Priscus Attalus, and that old Roman engaged him in earnest conversation—the sound of the great horn still ringing in his head—he heard an intimation in the old man's words that chafed a sore wound in his pride.

"The Emperor will soon know you're here," Priscus Attalus said, "if he doesn't already."

Atawulf glanced sideways at the old Roman. "I mean him to."

"Do you? Is that wise?"

"We're not hiding. Do you think we're hiding, Priscus Attalus?"

"Why . . . I . . . naturally I assumed . . ."

"Like rabbits run to our holes?"

"Well . . ." The old statesman, embarrassed, clearly believed that had been the Goths' purpose in disappearing into the great warren that was the villa.

And it irked Atawulf that the Roman was half-right. They had needed this safe haven, this sanctuary, needed it desperately in the beginning. But now the people were healing, their strength and spirit reviving, reappearing like the spring buds on these bare trees, a hazy hint of green, promising life, promising everything.

He mulled over his thoughts, staring up at the gnarled, greening limbs. Abruptly he shot a sharp look at Priscus Attalus.

"Do you think Honorius believes we are *hiding*? A day's ride from Rome?"

"Honorius believes what his officials tell him to believe."

"If he thinks we hide here from his legions, I'll let him know otherwise. Priscus, write me a message to the Emperor—something official and pompous. Inform him that we occupy Hadrian's Villa, at our leisure, and that if he objects he may come and evict us."

"For what purpose shall I say you are here, Your Majesty?"

"Purpose? Bile in his spleen? Poison in his dreams? Purpose enough, Priscus." The king clapped the former Senator's narrow shoulder. "But I take your meaning. If we seem to have some strategy, preferably something sticky and annoying, the Emperor and his officials will have a gleeful time countering it. We'll come up with something that'll keep them so busy trying to get around it, they'll never get around to *doing* anything about it—or us."

"I must admit, Your Majesty, that such a simple ruse might accomplish that end . . ."

"Of course it will. Alaric always said offering outrageous terms works no end of havoc with Romans."

Priscus Attalus sighed. "I blush to agree. What outrageous terms shall I put to the Emperor?"

"Well, let's see." Musingly Atawulf gazed into the endless blue overhead. "We can't just repeat all our usual demands—they're ready for those—and we can't expect any ransom for the Imperial Princess—they obviously hold her life of little account, though you would think her brother might at least *pretend* a little eagerness to have her back. She is, after all, the daughter of Theodosius and granddaughter of Valentinian, as Her Modesty has pointed out once or—" Now he spun abruptly upon Attalus. "The blood of emperors, Priscus! Born in the purple! Direct line to the throne! What sort of fool of an Emperor would dare let me keep her? Ah, ha-ha!"

Now he clapped both of Attalus's bony shoulders, jarring the older man.

"That's it, Priscus! Honorius has no heirs! That's it! Draft a proposal to the Emperor, stretch it with all the fancy braying and cackling you know, make it as confusing and pompous as you wish—aye, the more complicated, the better—but inform the Emperor that Atawulf proposes to marry his sister."

"He'll never agree." Priscus Attalus revealed not a flicker of surprise. In fact, he had often wondered how long Atawulf would take to discover what he himself had known weeks ago—that the King of the Goths and the Imperial Princess were two rich and wildly diverse wines, a spicy, heady blend, potent and potentially dangerous, but too tempting not to mix.

"Naturally, he'll not agree, but he'll have to wrest with the worrisome possibility that *I* might sire the only direct heirs to the Western throne—and the next Emperor might be half-Goth." Atawulf grinned gleefully, imagining Honorius's discomfort.

"Now, let me think . . ." He leaned indolently against the

bole of a tree, scratched his beard, then squinted thoughtfully up at the glint of sun dazzling off one of the grand balconies overlooking the Vale of Time.

"We have been supplicants to the Empire for too long, Priscus," he said suddenly. "Write me a proposal between equal sovereigns, a treaty between nations. Put to the Emperor terms of marriage between royal houses. On our part we will provide the throne with strong heirs, we will add the strength and arms of the Goths to that of the Empire, and for all time our purposes and those of the Roman Empire will be the same. On his part the Emperor will cede to the Goths good, fertile land, which lands to be mutually agreed upon by both parties. The Imperial Princess, of course, will retain ownership and profit from all lands and properties which she inherited from the royal lines of Theodosius and Valentinian."

"Oh, he won't like that; the princess owns properties in some of the richest provinces in the Empire."

"Ah, and while she's hostage those properties are administered by the Emperor. And when she marries . . ."

"They are all hers."

"But if she dies with no heirs . . . ?"

"They belong to the Empire."

"You don't suppose, do you, that Honorius has been *hoping* we'd murder his sister?"

"Half sister," corrected Priscus, "but no, I'd not imagine such infamy of Honorius, but his advisors at court may be anxious to swell the Imperial coffers."

"Won't a *marriage* make them cluck and cackle like a lot of worried hens! But we don't want to make them hasty. Add a few annoying terms, such as, oh, the Goths retaining the right to make treaties with other nations, or the right to draw up our own laws, or the right to veto Imperial edicts—terms they'll find excuses to haggle over—so they can stall us."

"Stall us, Your Majesty?"

"Naturally, Priscus, we want them to stall us."

"Naturally," echoed Priscus Attalus, momentarily confused, so caught up in the notion of a royal marriage.

"Have you forgotten? We know they're never going to consent, so we're stalling *them*. But they're not to realize that; they must believe they are stalling *us*. Therefore, you will hint—not threaten, but hint—that I'm only awaiting settlement of properties and terms out of diplomatic courtesy. Make them worry that if they reject my proposal out of hand, I might take royal offense, marry Galla Placidia without the Emperor's consent, and produce half-barbarian sons with better claim to the purple than any in the Empire."

Bold Wolf grinned at his own audacity. "Can you do that, Priscus Attalus?"

"Tricky, but I can do it. This will be a lengthy document..."

"The longer, the better. And brazen it up like an Imperial document—purple parchment, gold ink, the whole bit, bridle, and saddle."

"Do, um, you wish Princess Placidia's signature on this document?"

"No, no, that won't be necessary."

"I know the Imperial Princess well, Your Majesty. She will most assuredly take offense if you propose marriage without her consent."

"I'm sure of it," grinned Atawulf, "but what she doesn't know..."

"You can't be thinking of keeping this from her."

"What would you suggest? Her fever may be down, but she's as weak as a newborn babe, and I'm not of a mind to upset her."

"So you concede that she'll be upset when she finds out you're making secret arrangements to marry her."

"I thought you understood; the whole thing is a ruse; she need never know."

"Ah, that will make all the difference, Majesty. Should she

find out, she'll be happier to learn you are merely *using* her in a scheme to confound the Emperor."

"All right!" He paced on down the path. "I'll tell her!" Then he spun and paced back, pointing a warning at the old man. "But I'll choose the time."

"A judicious time, I hope, Majesty."

Atawulf stared up at the grand balcony, from which colorful woolen skirts and tunics hung drying in the sun.

"Right."

Dia believed she was going to die, and she didn't care. For days, seeming more like weeks, she prayed for respite, any respite from this wretched fever, and if it had to be death, let it get on with it.

She could no longer remember a time without blinding headache, terrible thirst, and raw, burning throat. Suffocating and sweating one moment, freezing and shaking the next, her body racked her with cruelest torture. She could not rest, could not sit up, could not drink, could not swallow. Her limbs moved restlessly; they ached in every bone, and her flesh, where it chafed beneath the covers, prickled and shivered.

The headache made her cry, and the fever tormented her with chaotic nightmares, and she wished she were dead, really dead, and she told Thalia so, and Thalia merely said, "I know," and wrung cool droplets of water from a cloth onto her hot forehead.

She knew she should be praying to be well, but she had forgotten how it felt to be well; her whole world was reduced to a bed of misery.

Then the fever cooled, and her eyes didn't hurt any longer, and she swallowed cool water and it tasted clean and smooth going down. She still felt as if she'd been buried alive and dug up again, but the smell of the room was not so suffocating, the light not so blinding, the bed not so like a bed of nettles.

Thalia gave her warm broth to drink, and she discovered she

was hungry. She managed a wraith-like smile for Thalia and Chrysanthia. She became cross and demanding, and Chrysanthia told her that she was not the first nor the last person to live through a fever, so she could stop being such a baby about it. Thalia just shook her head and said she was glad Miss Dia felt well enough to be snappish, and Dia, feeling abused, sulked. She turned over in bed, her back to them, and wept quietly, until Thalia leaned over and kissed her forehead and sat humming her to sleep.

Singing woke her, the full-throated chirping of a thrush outside her window, and the thrush song trilled on and on in jubilant announcement of a fine spring morning.

She surprised herself by laughing at the sound.

Soon the trees below her balcony window hosted a spectrum of songbirds, and the songs made her smile. Two days later she was allowed to sit out on the balcony, her couch warm in the afternoon sun, and she could see the trees bursting with buds.

She felt newborn. Everything was a delight to her. Since that wretched, miserable sickness had lifted, her senses tingled with life. Sensations she scarcely noticed before were now an experience of pure pleasure, like the heat of the sun on her face, the brush of a breeze upon her arms, wisps of hair tickling the back of her neck and making her laugh.

She found new delight in hot, steaming bread and sharp cheese and watered wine, and the smell of pine-scented oil burning in the lamps. She loved the sound of children's laughter, and the sound of flute; sometimes at evensong a solitary player pierced the cool air with beauty. She loved how the sun struck and flamed to glowing bronze the red roof of the round pavilion beyond the garden.

Ah, the garden. *Her* garden. It lay just below her balcony, the most private balcony in the villa, facing not inward to the peristyle, but outward from the Imperial bedroom over the most private little garden in the villa.

Rousing from its winter nap, the sleepy little garden peeked out into spring with green shoots and buds and tiny yellow flowers hiding in the old grass. Insects crawled beneath winter vegetation and birds hopped down from branches to snatch them up. Within days, it seemed, the garden was alive with birds singing and courting and nest building, and rich with the delicious smell of earth basking in sunshine.

She found herself murmuring a prayer of thanks every day just for being alive and feeling well and having so much life around her to enjoy.

From her chambers she could smell the pungent odor of horses in the peristyle, and even this delighted her. She ventured from her rooms out onto the inner balcony, which faced the peristyle, where she leaned over the balustrade to fill her senses with the presence of animal life. She watched the horses, their coats shining in the sun, and smiled as she pictured Atawulf herding his dusty war-horses into the Imperial peristyle as though it were a frontier post.

People on the inner balconies greeted her with waves and smiles and good-mornings, and she found herself smiling and nodding back at them. Soon she had visitors. When she was ill, she had been vaguely aware that Singledia and Winnifreya often stopped in to see how she fared, and now those two women came up to her balcony to visit. She invited them to dinner next evening, and they dined in the sun on Dia's garden balcony.

And her new awareness extended to the eyes and expressions of people, and she saw starkly the grief deepening Winn's countenance, and how the absence of Alaric in her life had taken the light out of her eyes. And her heart ached for Winnifreya, and it grieved her that she could do nothing to ease such loneliness.

Singledia the Younger slipped in to visit. Thalia had just washed Dia's hair and was brushing it in the sun until it shone dark amber and shimmering brown, and Singledia begged to be allowed to braid it. Neither woman had the heart to refuse, for the girl's own blond tresses had gone to the grave with her father, and her golden locks were too short for braiding.

Always there was Thalia. Patient, constant Thalia, with grave countenance and smiling jet eyes. Thalia, who with deft, gentle hands had bathed her, dressed her, fed her, even helped her to the chamber pot when she was dizzy and weak. Thalia, who soothed and hummed, and scolded scarcely at all, even when Dia had been a wretched tyrant.

Thalia, who knew the best and worst of her, and loved her for both.

Thalia, whom she had almost lost, whom she never, ever wanted to contemplate losing.

She surprised Thalia with an impulsive hug one afternoon and cajoled her to stop fussing with things and come sit out on the balcony and enjoy the fine day. Thalia let fall the silk coverlet she had billowed over the bed, shot Dia a droll look from beneath black lashes, and warned Dia she would soon spoil her poor handmaiden so that she'd be no good for anything. At which Dia laughed and countered that she was already spoiled, and she might as well come out and take advantage of it; so the two of them traipsed out upon the balcony, letting the balmy breeze play in their hair and the happy shouts of children draw them to the balustrade.

In the private little garden below, *her* garden, children dashed about, playing a game of hide and chase, and for a moment Dia felt a twinge of annoyance that her special place had been invaded. Then she smiled, remembering what it had been like running through the villa when she and Thalia were little girls. Nothing was safe from the curiosity of children, born explorers, and likely the children felt the garden was *their* special place, *their* secret. Suddenly it seemed right, these children of the Goths, these wandering, homeless children filling the old villa with giggles and shouts, for what would a spring day be without children?

She saw Atawulf's children among them, Athelwulf and Amalasuntha, and when the little girl glanced up, Dia waved. Hesitantly the child waved back, but dashed quickly away beneath the bright new foliage.

She told Thalia she despaired of winning Atawulf's children

over, for she had never paid the slightest attention to children and knew so little about them. Thalia raised the black wings of her brows. Atawulf again.

Dia and Thalia spent the afternoon recalling the many summers of their childhood spent in this magical villa, or so the beautiful rambling labyrinth of walks and gardens and hidden temples had seemed to them then. And yes, it still felt magical, they agreed, with a sense of quiet, of harmony, of peace that bathed the soul with contentment.

And every day there was Chrysanthia bustling in and out, a ball of purposeful busyness, defying the natural laws of old age.

Dia insisted she felt well enough to stroll down to the Emperor's private baths, which, as the days warmed, had been vacated by restless Goths well-recovered and eager to be out in fresh, cool air. Thalia accompanied her to the bathhouse with the great round sunroom.

Then, after the rubdown, after Thalia had massaged her body with almond-scented oil and scraped her clean with the strigil, Dia relaxed in the hot pool, soaking every vestige of the illness from her pores.

"Oh, Thalia, this is heavenly. I do believe I'd forgotten what a real bath feels like."

"I know *I* have," Thalia agreed wholeheartedly.

"Well, goodness, get into the pool. I simply had to have a rubdown and scraping as only you can do them, as only can be properly done in a steaming bathhouse." She leaned her head against the side of the pool and sighed.

"I think I shall never leave civilization again, Thalia."

Thalia rippled the water happily. "I hope you're right."

"Oh, I am. You watch, dear girl. I intend to see that we are not dragged tired, dirty, and hungry from one end of the Empire to the other like vagabonds. We're home, and somehow we'll stay home."

"And what about His Majesty King Goth, miss?"

"Atawulf hasn't a prayer. I feel I could fly from the top of the walls today."

Thalia laughed. "Thank goodness! I thought you'd never feel your old self again, Mistress Dia."

"I'm *more* than my old self," she said, eyes reflecting the dancing surface of the water. "Everything feels wonderful, exquisite, as though I'd never felt it before. This heavenly warm bath, the echoes you made when you laughed just now, sunlight dancing on the water—why, just this morning the mere shape of a white cloud against blue sky gave me shivers right down to my soul. I can't really explain it . . ."

Thalia answered seriously. "I think I know, miss. I believe I feel more *alive* than before . . . before I fell ill. Everything seems . . . sharper. Something about being so close to death . . ."

"Yes, feeling *alive!* Thalia, that's it. It's feeling alive again, and being grateful for every moment, appreciating life, and everything that's good about it . . . and everyone."

Thalia raised her eyebrows. "Everyone, miss?"

"Yes, why not everyone?"

"Why not indeed?" She had been about to say, "Even Atawulf?" but she changed her mind. It was none of her business; let fate take its natural course. "I hope you're including your poor handmaiden, Mistress Dia."

Dia laughed. "You're incorrigible, Thalia. Yes, especially my poor handmaiden, who has become absolutely too spoiled for her own good."

She and Thalia spent the cooler mornings in the Emperor's sitting room playing at tables, perfume wafting from scented bowls to merge with the odor of horses from the peristyle. The spacious, airy room itself was curtained with sheer rose silk, and the floor patterned like a flower garden. The furnishings, of burnished gold and rich polished woods, were elegant, tasteful, and practical.

There was ever a wine cart at hand, and a refreshment cart loaded with platters of cheeses, dried figs and apricots, and honeyed pastries. Usually a young, dandy-curled boy plucked upon a lyre in the corner. Sometimes Chrysanthia sat with them and chattered, and often Rayard lurked in the doorway, even though Dia chided him for thinking she needed guarding in her own villa. She and Thalia sat at the game table with its inlaid squares of cherrywood and black walnut and played with game pieces of gold and obsidian.

And one day, suddenly, there was Atawulf, stepping into her sitting room, startling her unduly, for there was no reason for her to feel flustered, nor for her heart to beat wildly. To hide the slow blush she felt creeping up her cheeks she stood abruptly and knocked awry the table. Game pieces rolled across the floral mosaic beneath their feet.

Breathlessly she greeted him. He had been absent from the villa for several days, but she knew from Thalia that he had come by to inquire about her every evening when she was ill.

"Well, Your Royalty, you're looking . . ." *Beautiful,* he wanted to say, but he finished lamely with "well."

"I *am* well," she answered, "and I thank you for your concern. Thalia tells me you've asked about my health. I'm happy to report that I've been up and about for several days now."

"I've been away," he excused himself quickly. "For nearly a week."

"I know. Very little passes in the villa that Chrysanthia does not tell us." She took a deep breath; the issue could not be avoided. "I suppose you've been raiding the countryside."

"Umbria." He could be as blunt as she. "I've been pillaging Umbria."

"I have relations in Umbria, aunts who are very dear to me."

His blue eyes had fixed upon a fallen obsidian game piece; he rolled it back and forth beneath his dusty, hob-nailed boot. He had neither changed clothes nor eaten, but come straight to see for himself how she fared, straight from raiding her people, as though he had only been out hunting. What had he been thinking?

The blue eyes glimmered at her beneath golden hawk-brows.

"I've not been killing your people, if that's what you fear. Nor will I, unless they be fools enough to attack me. Nor am I burning the fields and villages behind me. That was a hard lesson learned; without the land and the people there is no next harvest should we need it."

"Without the harvest my people will starve."

"Let the Emperor see to them."

She turned away and with sudden absorption began helping Thalia retrieve the game pieces. The Emperor, she knew well, would let them starve; let the Goths deplete every resource until they were forced to move on, no matter the cost to the Roman people.

At this moment, Priscus Attalus was announced by a slave. The old statesman bowed himself into her presence, but when he raised his bald head his grey-eyed glance jumped from Atawulf to Dia and then sharply back to Atawulf.

Atawulf shifted from foot to foot, flushed, and looking at no one, hastily took his leave with a mumbled, "The horses need rubbing down. Hard ride." And he was gone.

Dia looked inquiringly at Priscus Attalus, but that man fared no better. He stood staring at the princess, working his mouth noiselessly. At last he snapped it shut.

"Nobilissima."

"Yes. Correct, Priscus."

"My pardons . . ."

"Pardons for what, Priscus?"

"Why—what a fool I am—I've forgotten why I came! I'm an old man, Princess, and it seems . . . well, if you'll please forgive me . . ."

Priscus Attalus retreated so quickly he forgot to bow. Dia turned wide turquoise eyes on Thalia.

"What do you suppose that was all about?"

• • •

Priscus Attalus, huffing with exertion, caught up with Atawulf as the king led his black war-horse into the huge courtyard surrounding the great swimming pool. He halted beside man and horse, unable to force words from his gasping lungs.

Atawulf slid the dusty red saddle off the black and flung it over a marble bench. The colonnaded courtyard was milling with horses and men, and a brown cloud of dust stirred up by hooves coated everything; even the water in the pool was brown.

Priscus Attalus had time to regret the loss of the lawn; any hope of spring grass was stamped and pawed out of the soil. His sandaled feet deftly avoided both horse dung and hooves. King Atawulf pointedly ignored him, his attention on rubbing down his horse. The old man puffed out his annoyance.

"You didn't tell her!"

"I haven't had a chance."

"You're not going to tell her."

"I am."

"But you didn't."

"You interrupted."

"You ran."

"I did not run."

"Sprinted, in fact."

"Priscus!" growled the King of the Goths. "You harry me at your peril."

"Peril? It seems to me, Majesty, the only peril here is yours. The peril of dealing falsely with the Imperial Princess."

The black war-horse snorted and looked back to ascertain just what the holdup was on his rubdown. Atawulf returned to the task.

"That's my problem," he told Priscus.

"On the contrary, it is mine. She'll never trust me again."

"She doesn't trust you now, you old fox."

The former Prefect squared his shoulders stubbornly, thrust his chin at the barbarian.

"I beg to differ, Majesty. Princess Placidia trusts me absolutely."

"Does she now?"

"I hate to deceive her."

"We're not deceiving her, Priscus. The time is not right."

"I fail to see what difference . . ."

"Ah, therein lies the difference."

"Majesty?"

"You fail to see. I see perfectly. Now, if you will pardon me, I have only three things—no, four things—on my mind. My horse, a colossal dinner, an hour in the bath, and a month's sleep."

"But Majesty . . ."

"Go!"

Priscus Attalus pressed his lips together in annoyance, but departed without further argument, to Atawulf's relief. Aye, Atawulf saw perfectly, all right. He had mulled on it much, these days and nights he had been raiding. How important was the land! Good earth was life and nurture, and more than ever he was determined that his people would have land of their own.

Never could they find peace if they were forever wandering, never prosper without homes and crops and pastures—fertile soil and water, wood for shelter and fire. Free as the wind they were, but they could not live on air alone!

He needed an alliance with Ravenna, with the Emperor, much as it galled him to admit it. And the best alliance he had already proposed. He had sent that offer to buy time, buy negotiation instead of retaliation, but now . . . now . . .

She'll never agree. What makes you think she's going to agree?

I'll worry about that when I have to.

11

D<small>IA FOUND</small> herself in the peculiar position of defending Atawulf. Chrysanthia harrumphed and clucked and said, "King? Robber King, if you ask me."

"Chrysanthia, no one asked you. You know nothing of the matter . . . of what it's like to be responsible for a whole nation. Atawulf is feeding his people, which is what any good king should be doing. He does all he can for the succor of his people; I wish I could say as much for the Emperor." She shook her head in disbelief. "My brother . . . abandoning the people like this . . ."

Suddenly Princess Placidia smiled, transforming her face into kindness. She really did not wish to deflate the old woman, merely to set her straight.

"Have I told you, Chrysanthia," Dia said brightly, "I truly couldn't do without you? You're a treasure, putting up thirty thousand Goths in a trifling and keeping everything running so smoothly. Why, the baths were even hot. And I believe that's what

I'd like more than anything right now, a long, luxurious soak. Thalia, gather our things and some sweet-smelling oils for the water—rose and hyacinth, I think."

As Placidia rose to go, Chrysanthia opened her mouth as though to speak, but snapped it shut again immediately. What she had to say could be said without impertinence, but she resolved to hold her tongue about this, too: she happened to know that King Atawulf had a habit of bathing in the Emperor's private bathhouse whenever he returned from a long ride. He was just as likely bathing now as not, and Chrysanthia regretted only that she could not be there to see what a scene their meeting might create.

So the two women, princess and handmaiden, strolled through the little garden, past the round island pavilion, and into Hadrian's bathhouse with the great round sunroom and hot and warm pools. The marbled room was hot and steamy already, with billowing fog making the air hazy and damp. Thalia carried a small basket of scents and oils and strigils, and over her arm were draped two large towels of brushed white linen.

As they halted near the marble rim of the hottest bath, its shadowed corners obscured by steam, a towel slipped from Thalia's arm and fell in a heap on the wet tiles. Dia bent to rescue it, but as her fingers closed on the cloth, a sound froze her.

The most awful, horrible animal sound she had ever heard, and she thought at once of a great bear lurking in the water just below her feet, for as a child her vivid imagination had often struck upon the notion that Grandfather Valentinian's infamous bears must live somewhere about the villa. The forgotten, but undimmed suspicion resurfaced.

She heard it again, that inhuman snarling, and flung the towel straight down upon a movement in the water below. To her terror, with snorts and snarls and splashes, the creature burst from the water, man-high, a towering, thrashing beast beneath the wet towel.

With a shriek, Dia staggered backward into Thalia.
"*A bear!*"

Atawulf didn't remember falling asleep, didn't remember where he was, but he knew he was being drowned. When the cloth fell over his face, startling him awake and causing him to strike his head hard on marble, he didn't realize he was in water until it closed over his head.

Roaring, he shot to his feet, the now sopping material clinging around his arms and covering his mouth and nose and eyes.

As Dia staggered against her, Thalia screamed and flung her basket at the enraged creature. The basket struck it roundly in the face—she hoped it was the face—and the two women stumbled across the slippery floor.

"Assassins!" roared the creature, but to the women it was an unintelligible sputtering.

Struck in the face by an unknown assailant, Atawulf was sure he was under attack. Hip-deep in water, he fought the clinging material and tried to stride forward. His big toe struck a submerged step, hard.

"Ouwwooo!"

Something about that howl sounded awfully familiar to Dia. She stopped and looked back just in time to see Atawulf, King of the Goths, claw the sopping towel from his face. The great head of tawny hair shook droplets in all directions.

Dia stood, hand over her mouth, her eyes glistening seas of mirth.

Atawulf's hawk-brows swooped at each other, his eyes a blue thunderstorm.

"*Woman, are you trying to drown me?*"

Dia's shoulders shook; she burst into gales and giggles of laughter.

"Oh!" she gasped. "I thought you were . . . a *bear!* You

looked . . . you looked so . . . *enraged!*" The thought of his angry bellows struck her as doubly funny; helplessly she clutched her sides and spun in a circle, laughing fit to choke.

"I'm sure you find it amusing to accost a man in the midst of a hard-earned nap and a much-deserved bath—accost him, half-drown him, throw . . . what's this? . . . *perfume* in his water! . . . and then laugh at him."

Dia, having nearly regained her composure, dissolved into gleeful shrieks again.

"Is this," Atawulf drawled, "what royal ladies do for amusement? Surprise naked men in the bath?" A broad grin split his dripping beard. "Or is this some blue-blood mating ritual—I hope?"

Dia giggled, but her eyes widened and fastened on the man standing in the water, his long hair dripping over broad glistening shoulders, fine chest hairs plastered to his rock-hard torso, flat abdomen moving powerfully with each breath, fists propped on the narrow of his hips, just where the rippling water was lapping at his pelvis.

Dia was breathlessly aware that he was perfectly nude, shockingly aware of just which part of his anatomy must be hidden just below the water's rippling surface. She shocked herself still more by not only looking, but actually feeling disappointment when all that was visible was the reflection of his upper body floating on the water.

Atawulf followed her gaze and grinned even more broadly, wolfishly, in fact. "Why, Your Royal Primness, whatever are you looking for?"

Dia went scarlet.

"Lose something?" Atawulf peered into his reflection.

"No! Yes! Our . . . our perfume vials."

Atawulf wrinkled his nose over the water. "Woman, you've fumigated my bath with flowers."

"*Your* bath? You've shed your grime in *my* bath, sir."

"Ha!"

"These are the private Imperial baths," Dia informed him in that maddeningly imperious tone of hers.

"Are they now?" said Atawulf softly. "And you'd like me to vacate them, I'll bet."

"Immediately."

"Charmed to, madam." Atawulf took a step toward her.

"You would not dare."

Atawulf put one foot onto the first underwater stair step.

"Thalia, we're leaving." She tugged Thalia by the arm and started for the door. Behind them she heard the unmistakable sound of a body rising from water. She resisted looking back and affected a dignified exit from the bath—dignified until she heard the unmistakable sound of bare feet slapping marble, then, with quickened steps, she hurried Thalia out the door.

Behind them they heard Atawulf's shout. "The bath's all yours, Your Royalty! 'Tis not so grimed as all that!"

They departed to the infuriating sound of deep-chested guffaws.

And when Bold Wolf, on his way to his long-anticipated soft bed, met his mother in the apartments, Singledia embraced the son she had not seen since he left for a week's foraging. She sniffed and leaned back to eye him suspiciously.

"You smell like roses. Going courting?"

"No, Ma, where do you get these notions?" Bold Wolf slipped through her grasp and sidled into the bedroom.

Her grey-blue eyes followed her son until he rolled onto the nearest bed with a contented groan.

"You told my *mother?*" Atawulf fairly shouted at the old man.

Priscus Attalus flinched but did not back down. "I had to, Majesty!"

"Of all people! I commanded you to tell no one about the

proposal, and the first thing you do is run straight to my own mother . . ."

"She *made* me tell her!"

"What? Am I to believe my mother tortured you?"

"She kept asking questions and guessing. She's a very good guesser, Majesty."

Atawulf shook his head in defeat. Even he would be hard put to hold out under Singledia's sharp eye and sharper tongue.

"Maybe she'll stay out of it," he muttered, casting a hopeful glance toward Heaven.

"Speaking of the proposal," ventured Priscus Attalus, "when are you going to tell Princess Placidia? Every moment I spend in her presence without telling her, I am lying through my silence. The sooner she's told, the better for my conscience—and nerves."

" 'Twill take a little longer than I thought."

"No, don't say this! Why?"

"Because I've changed my mind, Priscus, old fellow." Atawulf glanced over both his shoulders and leaned in to speak close to the man's wrinkled ear. "I'm going to marry her."

The old statesman sighed, his patience stretched thin. "Then you'll eventually have to bring the subject up, Majesty."

"There's no need for sarcasm; I know what I'm doing. A woman needs to be warmed up to the idea first."

"All diplomatic marriages are approached with the utmost decorum . . ."

"Aye, and I'm sure they're all tedious. But if I know Dia . . . Her Royalty will take righteous offense at being proposed to *diplomatically.*"

"Nonsense. That's how it's done."

"Priscus, how many women have you courted?"

"None. My marriage was arranged."

"Trust me. I know what I'm doing."

• • •

Spring settled in with all her glory, as though she had only just been away for a day, and now she trimmed the walks with greenery and bright pink and purple flowers nodding in yellow sunshine.

Tree branches budded so thickly and lushly, they seemed clothed in velvety green moss. A warm spring breeze caught Dia's hair and set it dancing.

She scampered down the stone steps from her balcony into the private little garden. Thalia tripped along behind her, and they followed the narrow path through the garden toward an open-air portico with a columned roof. And beyond the portico lay the little circular moat and its tiny island, and on the island was the round pavilion, its roof supported by rows of exquisite columns arranged in fluid lines curving inward, drawing their eyes and their footsteps ever inward into the center of the airy pavilion.

It was just as she remembered it. One of the movable bridges spanned the blue water that reflected the bright-blue paint of the moat, and she and Thalia trotted across the bridge and into the rippling sun-shadows patterning the floor of the pavilion, patterning their faces, arms, and dresses. Sunlight flooded through the center hole of the roof and defined the lines and curves and columns in light and dark, white and black, flashing across their eyelids as they spun across the floor.

Laughing and dizzy, they strolled back across the bridge, underneath the portico, and out into the narrow garden. They found buds near to bursting open, promising color and perfume, and tiny green leaves quivering in the bright air. The grass glowed emerald in the afternoon and felt cool beneath their bare feet, for they had shucked their sandals and were enjoying its delicious softness.

Bees hummed and buzzed, searching for early-blooming flowers, and birds chorused to each other in dulcet voices.

"Thalia, let's go to the end of the garden, to the crack in the wall and look out over the hills."

Through the tangled brush at the back of the garden they

went, stepping gingerly; vines thick as ropes crisscrossed the wall, but the great crack in the stones showed clear sky beyond. At least, it had seemed a great crack when they were children, when they had placed their small feet in the narrow split and hauled themselves up with vines to stand one behind the other in the widest part of the crack.

Dia put one foot in the split and grasped at vines. "I'm going up." She pulled herself upright against the wall. The crack seemed much smaller than it used to. To crawl into it she had to bend over and go headfirst. "There's only room for one. In fact, there's scarcely room for . . . *oh!*"

Her hand slipped, scraping down the stone, landing her sharply on her knee. She scrabbled for a foothold and her foot slipped, too. With a surprised gasp she slid abruptly into the crack.

"Are you all right, Miss Dia?" came Thalia's anxious voice.

"Yes, I'm fine. I'm just trying to get my hand free so I—there!" She tried to inch forward and push her midriff up from the split, but she managed somehow just to wedge herself deeper. No matter how she twisted and turned, she could not budge from that crack.

"Thalia, I think I'm stuck!"

"What? Oh, are you sure?"

"Of course I'm sure! Thalia, I can't move! Help me out of here!"

She was answered with silence behind her. Lingering silence.

"Thalia, if you are laughing at me you can just stop it. This is *not* funny!"

"Yesss . . . miss." Thalia fluttered around behind her, giving a tentative tug to one bare leg.

"Ow! Not that way, you goose! You can't pull me out; you'll have to lift me."

"How? I'll have to have help, miss."

"Then *find* someone. I *hate* this. I want out of here—*immedi-*

ately!" Dia's voice broke a little; she did not know if she was laughing or crying.

"I'm going—don't worry—I'll find someone! Stay right where you are, miss!"

Dia rolled her eyes. "Stay where you are, she says! Where does she imagine . . . Thalia! Wait! I forbid you to tell anyone but Chrysanthia—especially not . . . well, anyone. Do you hear me?"

She struggled briefly to free herself, but she was securely stuck from knee to neck. Her head hung out the other side of the wall, where she could see straight down to the low brush below. She turned her head from side to side, hoping to see no one who could see *her*.

Praying *he* would not find her like this, making an absolute fool of herself—again.

She laughed weakly to herself. This was just too absurd. Too embarrassing. Too typically Galla Placidia. How did she get into these predicaments?

Naturally, Thalia brought Atawulf to rescue her. Her handmaiden had come across him at the royal apartments, dropping by for a visit, and his disappointment at not finding Dia at home quickly turned into merriment as he followed the excited handmaiden and heard the story in fits and starts.

When he finally reached the wall, the sight was all he had anticipated. He stood back to savor it, with a grin that stretched his beard from ear to ear. And what an eyeful! That pert little rump hiked up in the air, and legs bare up to high thigh, shapely legs and dainty bare feet flailing haplessly in mid-air.

"Hah-Hoo!" he whooped, and exploded into shouts of pure glee.

"Oh, no!" Dia closed her eyes, mortified.

Atawulf stomped one foot, unable to breathe.

"Stop it!"

Atawulf roared until he wept.

Dia knotted her free fist and beat ineffectively on the stone.

Atawulf gasped. Finally his guffaws dwindled to chuckles and occasional sighs of disbelief.

"Oh, boy! Good—*ha!*—good afternoon, Your—ah—ha-*hah!*—Your—"

Dia waited impatiently until he stopped to catch his breath. "If you have quite finished laughing at me, kindly give me a hand down from here."

"Oh, charmed, Your Dignity. Now, don't get up. Don't stand on ceremony on my account."

"Don't you dare make fun of me!" Dia's voice was close to sputtering. "When you find someone in a difficult position, you've no need to humiliate that person even further."

"Aye, this is what I'd call a difficult position, all right. Certainly makes an interesting view from here."

"How dare you stare at my . . . my view!"

"Hard to miss."

"I demand that you help me down from here this instant!"

"Oh, you demand, do you?"

She bit her lip. Bit back an angry retort.

"Please!" she beseeched him with all the meekness at her command.

"What? I didn't quite catch that."

"Please!"

"Could you put a little honey in your voice, just for me?"

"Beast!" But she laughed.

Atawulf stepped up to the wall and studied her predicament. Shaking his head, he prepared to wriggle one hand beneath her midriff and the other beneath her thighs.

"Aah! What do you think you're doing?"

"Looking for a good handhold."

"That's my . . . get your hand away from my . . . bosom!"

"Hold still or I'll lose my grip. Ready?" His arms bulged as he lifted her straight up, scraping her between the stones, and pulled her backward against him, encircled in his arms. As he set her down her soft curves pressed warmly against him.

The effect on Atawulf was immediate and intense; reluctantly he let her pull away. She looked anywhere but at him, flustered and blushing and suddenly preoccupied with her scraped knee.

"I . . . thank you. I was quite . . . caught. I suppose I must seem . . ."

He waited. She resigned herself to going on.

". . . rather silly."

"*Uncanny* is the word that comes to mind. What in God's name were you doing crawling through the wall like a . . . no, don't tell me. This was another one of your escape attempts, no doubt."

"Certainly not. I climbed up to look at the . . . view." She admitted the last word reluctantly; her flesh still tingled where she had felt him through the soft material of her spring gown. This sudden awareness of the feel of his body she could not shake. Nor did she want to. She stood close enough to feel the heat of him, the life in him, and was sure he could feel the pulsing of her heart. She forced herself to step away, free of the powerful pull of him.

His blue eyes lifted from hers. "The view, eh?" Atawulf found a toehold, hoisted himself up and climbed by vine and stone all the way to the top of the wall. He stood upon the wall, leather-booted feet wide apart, bare arms akimbo, unshorn golden head bare to the wind.

"The view's fine! Come on up and have a look!" He knelt on the wall and reached down a hand to her.

Dia shook her head. "No, I . . . I couldn't."

"Why not?"

She wondered if she dared touch him ever again.

"Afraid, Your Royalty?"

Making up her mind quickly, she grasped the offered hand, and strong fingers closed about hers. Her toes scrambled roughly on the rock as Atawulf hauled her up to stand on the wall beside him.

Breathless, she gazed out over the countryside, which fell in lazy slopes from this remote wall of the villa. Pastures of new green lay like carpet below, and the landscape was artfully patterned with tree-lined avenues leading in all directions away from the villa. A flock of birds high in the shimmering blue wheeled in formation, and their wings flashed silver.

Dia breathed in the sky and let the wind play in her hair, and knew there never was a country as lovely as this anywhere else on Earth. Her country. Her Italia.

When she at last pulled her gaze from the glowing hills and trees and cloud-swept sky above, she discovered Atawulf watching her, eyes as blue as the sky they reflected.

He smiled down at her. She glowed in sunlight, amber and gold in her rich brown hair, flecks of green in her blue eyes, a fresh flush on her smooth cheeks as her face turned up to his.

"Truce?" he offered softly, the word rumbling.

She ventured a quick glance at him. "Truce," she agreed, turning her face again to the windswept vista.

"I'm hoping you'll show me your villa."

"Surely you've seen most of it already."

"But not through your eyes. You grew up here?"

"The happiest memories of my childhood are here. I came every year with my aunts—summers, usually, sometimes spring, too." She laughed and looked down at her feet, dirt-brown and stone-scraped. "This was the only place I was allowed to go barefoot, or dance in the rain, or climb trees. My aunties considered it an essential part of childhood."

"Wisely."

"Yes. Because of them the villa feels more like home to me than any of the Imperial palaces ever could. I feel . . . freer here." She turned and waved down at Thalia, who watched them from below. "Thalia and I claimed this garden for our own. In summer it has blackberries; we used to eat them right off the vine. And over there—my summer palace, I called it—the island pavilion. Have you been inside?"

"Aye, but only once. 'Tis little shelter from wind or rain . . ."

"That's because it's a sun palace. Come on, I'll show you."

She hesitated. "If you'll help me down."

He put out both broad hands. "Hold on; I'll lower you."

They came down from the wall, and with Thalia joining them, Dia led the way back to the island pavilion. There were nooks where cushioned couches provided cozy places for dining, for reading or sleeping; there were cabinets for scrolls and tables, and even a small latrine. But the large central space of the pavilion was open to the sky and consisted of little more than slender marble columns arrayed around a central fountain.

"This is where Hadrian came to read, or rest, or just think, away from the rest of the villa. See, when the bridges are drawn aside, the moat keeps out idle wanderers, and the slaves knew not to disturb him. He designed it himself, for solitude and for beauty. He designed the whole villa, really. If he hadn't been Emperor, he would have made a great architect."

"But he couldn't have built at his whim if he hadn't been Emperor. Only an Emperor could build a fantastic place like this."

"A dream palace, you mean?"

"Aye, and with little more substance than a dream."

"It isn't meant to have substance—only space and contour and light. See, as we move, the patterns of the columns move, making shifting planes and depths, yet the design is so simple. 'Simplicity through complexity,' my aunt Grata's architect used to say."

Atawulf thought that phrase could describe the whole rambling villa, each building its own work of art. Though many of the structures were practical, many seemed built for the sheer love of beauty.

"The view is everything, eh?" mused Atawulf, staring from the center of the pavilion through the north side, which was no more than a circle of columns. Beyond the columns he could see across the moat, through the nearby portico, and all the length of the garden to an old vine-choked shrine.

"Yes, yes, the view is everything." Dia nodded. "The villa seems a jumble of pools and colonnades and pavilions with no plan or design, until you realize each structure is arranged to catch the sun a certain way, or draw the summer breezes, or frame a lovely view."

"Aye. I've formed a few opinions of Hadrian since seeing his villa."

"Have you? Well, then, what has King Atawulf decided about Hadrian just from looking at his villa? Other than his genius, of course."

Atawulf, crossing the little footbridge, shot an amused glance in her direction. "Plenty. For one, he was a man who loved beautiful surroundings."

"Obviously."

"He was a meticulous planner—and observer. He imagined each structure as it would fit into the seasons—with the path of the sun and the habits of the winds. That takes a good eye for nature, and long study."

"Why, yes, it would," Dia agreed. "I hadn't thought of that."

"And he loved the sun. This little pavilion of his could as well be a temple to the sun."

"Yes, he worshipped Apollo."

"Naturally."

"You didn't say it."

"Too obvious. There are shrines everywhere." As they strolled around the perfectly circular blue moat, Atawulf waved back toward the wild little garden, irregularly shaped and seemingly unplanned.

"And he worshipped nature."

"He did not!"

"He loved it, at any rate. Understood it. Look how the buildings follow the coutours of the land, and look how trees and gardens are everywhere you turn."

They walked on around the island and through an archway in a surrounding wall. Stone steps led them eventually to the double-tiered colonnade, and upon reaching the upper level they strolled along the long covered walkway open at both sides to a cool breeze. To the north they could see far across the rolling pastureland with its stately avenues lined with great old trees. In hot summer those trees would afford welcome shade for riders galloping toward the wooded hills. To the south the colonnade looked down upon the great swimming pool and park, though now horses milled within the vast enclosure, raising dust and muck, and drank from the marble pool.

"There's your Red Demon!" Dia exclaimed with pleasure. "His legs are healed."

"Aye. I've been exercising him, but I'm riding the black now, until I'm sure Demon's ready."

Atawulf whistled piercingly, and the red stallion raised his head, ears forward, and drummed the dirt in a little dance at the sound of his master's whistle.

Dia turned to look out toward the oak-covered hills and endless sky, her hair tousled by the wind. "The breeze is warm even up here. This just had to be built for walking on perfect spring days like this."

Atawulf shook his head. " 'Tis for running, I'd say. Beginning at the Emperor's bath. One good run along the colonnade, then a turn at the end and back along the inside corridor, and a plunge back into the bath. You should try it—heats the blood, clears the lungs."

Dia half-smiled, imagining Atawulf, straight from the warm bath, sprinting all out along this high colonnade, and it occurred to her that he would be naked to the sun and air, bare legs flashing, muscles straining. She shook off the image.

"I think we should go down now," she announced. Belatedly she looked around for her maid. "Now where could Thalia have gotten off to?"

"I waved her on home. We don't need your shadow, Miss Prim and Proper."

"I wish you wouldn't call me that."

"Then what? Your Royalty?"

"No."

"Dia."

She turned. Her name rumbled intimate and warm from his lips. She remembered his tawny beard felt like soft fur . . . His eyes watched her, waiting.

She lowered her dark lashes. "Yes. Dia. I prefer it."

"So do I."

She walked quickly ahead of him down the marble steps. Why did his voice sound like a caress? Why did her every thought come back, inescapably, to the powerful physical sense of him?

She wondered what he felt when he looked at her, wondered if he could read her thoughts as clearly as she felt them burning her face.

And Atawulf, seeing her quick retreat, could only guess that he was pushing her—too fast and too far. If he didn't ease up she might run away altogether. Ah, a plague on princesses and their sheltered lives!

"Hadrian loved to walk," Atawulf observed abruptly. "He built covered walkways and paved paths everywhere."

"Yes, but he loved to walk in comfort, didn't he? You can walk almost anywhere in the villa sheltered from rain, or shaded from the sun when it's hot."

"And he loved water." Atawulf stared at the huge waterfall cascading down semicircular steps at the end of yet another long park. This park, like the others in the complex, now held a goodly number of their horses. "He liked running water. The *sound* of water."

"It's almost like a lullaby, isn't it? In summer I'd stay on the island and the water would sing me to sleep."

"Sometimes I forget it's there," he said, "and then suddenly I hear it. The sound is so constant, and soothing. I wonder . . . is that why this place seems so peaceful?"

"I think so."

Abruptly he turned to her, his eyes intent. "Dia, I never told you . . . never thanked you for guiding us to this place . . . for sharing this sanctuary with my people. We . . . they needed it."

"I never wished your people harm, Bold Wolf." Her gaze was steady. "I hope you believe that."

"Aye, I know. I was angry at the sea, at the world, at God—everything—and you were . . ." He almost said she was the thorn in his heart, how he was as much angry with himself for loving her.

"I was Roman," she said for him. "Imperial Roman."

"It seemed to matter then."

"But not now?"

"No. Not now."

Her heart fluttered, but she did not know what to say. Whether they were Roman or Goth did not matter here, now—but what of tomorrow, when he could as easily ride off raiding and pillaging her people, when the Goths could soon be sacking cities, burning homes . . . when the legions could be marching against this villa—which, no matter what her feelings were for these people and their king, she knew the legions should be doing.

Later that afternoon, she laughed when Atawulf insisted Hadrian liked the sound of his own voice, and he took her to the great dome to prove it. He howled into the dome, and then he cajoled her until she howled, too, and made it echo for her.

Too quickly the days streamed by, like the waters flowing around them. Spring flowered, and the rich earthen smell of growing things permeated their senses, the very air laden with life.

And the air sang. The waters chuckled, birds warbled, and honeybees hummed and hovered over dew-laden blooms, nuzzling their fuzzy heads in golden nectar until they were so rich with gold dust they could scarcely fly.

Some days the air was so still they could hear the delicate whirring of bird's wings swift overhead.

Halcyon days they were to Dia, peaceful and overflowing and

sensual, as though the world had come alive just for her. She knew her newborn delight was due to more than her recovery; she knew the feeling blossomed during those hours she spent in Atawulf's company. She looked forward to seeing him each day.

And he, finding excuses to remain at the villa, looked to the repairing of the Goths' weapons and shields, armor and saddles. Wallia he put in charge of travel readiness, repairs of wagons and harnesses, while Singledia and Winnifreya dealt with the mending of the tents and blankets and clothing. The King of the Goths made sure his men were war-ready, too, and joined them when they practiced swordplay and spear throwing.

As the pastures greened, Atawulf moved the frisky horses out of the villa proper and into the wide open meadows on the rolling slopes below. He drilled his cavalry before the walls, charging and wheeling and circling; the men put the horses through their paces and practiced striking each other's shields with lances or swords as they passed at lightning speed.

Bold Wolf commanded the finest cavalrymen who ever rode together, and he made sure they knew it, and lived up to it. He rode with them, usually on the black, but he rode Demon in some of the drills, and the red stallion's mane flew as he wheeled in tandem with the other horses, his head dipped, tail flashed, and he neighed his excitement and triumph.

And at the end of each day, Atawulf looked forward with light step and jubilant heart to his evening stroll with Placidia. She filled up his empty spaces, lightened his heart, and he felt he wanted things to never change. He wanted nothing more for his contentment than this radiant woman beside him, and if he put off revealing his feelings for her and asking her to be his wife, it was because he would also have to tell her about the proposal he had sent to her brother for an alliance, and he feared to rush her, feared to spoil this easy companionship between them. He treasured the peaceful moments they enjoyed together, but he knew he must speak; why then was he so reluctant?

Priscus Attalus reminded him frequently of his duty.

"You must tell her *now*," said the old statesman for the hundredth time. "You've courted long enough."

"Don't rush me," grinned Atawulf. "I'm just getting to the good part."

Priscus Attalus was not to be charmed or diverted. "No, I am truly sorry, Your Majesty, but I must not bend on this. I've gone too far already, compromising my integrity. My duty is to the Imperial Princess, and as her chief advisor and confidant . . ."

"You exaggerate, Priscus."

"I will not be put off." Attalus looked as stern as Atawulf had ever seen him. "I regret that it has come to this, Majesty, but I will be forced to inform her myself if you will not."

Atawulf stared at him, eyes narrowed in his most ferocious glare, but Priscus Attalus stood his ground, swallowing once nervously.

"Is this a *threat*, Priscus?" Atawulf dared him.

"Forgive me, but, yes."

"Ha!" Atawulf beat his fists together and stomped away and back again. "You are the goddamnedest, stubbornest, most cantankerous old goat I've ever seen! You would do it, too, wouldn't you!"

They stood glaring, the barbarian looming over the old man by half a head, each determined to stare the other down.

"All right!" growled Atawulf. He jabbed a finger in Attalus's determined face. "You win! We'll try it your way. You'd better be right."

"Splendid! Of course I'm right." Priscus Attalus beamed and talked enthusiastically. "Now, I've thought it all out and come up with a marvelous plan. You'll invite Galla Placidia to dine with you, somewhere private and cozy, somewhere romantic. A little wine, a compliment or two, and then you'll tell her about the proposal and declare your love straightforwardly and honestly."

Atawulf stared at Priscus in unfeigned surprise. Then the King of the Goths grinned and draped a brawny arm around the thin old shoulders.

"Priscus Attalus, I've greatly misjudged you, I see. If you took to courting, you'd have every eligible noblewoman in the Empire lining up at your door."

King Atawulf respectfully requested Princess Placidia's company for the afternoon and an early dinner.

Princess Placidia most graciously accepted, and with flushed excitement sent Chrysanthia and Thalia flying to help her get ready. Thalia brushed her hair until it shone, then put it up for her, piling her autumn-brown tresses in cascading curls.

At the last moment Dia changed her mind and decided to forgo the beaded jewels Thalia had draped upon her head. Instead she sent her maid out to gather flowers, purple and pale blue and rosy pink, and Thalia wove them into a garland to wear in her hair.

She did wear a simple strand of blue topaz and silver; and earrings, little sparkling droplets of blue; and a slender bracelet of the same. Nestled in the cleft of her breasts she wore the tiny locket that held her mother's portrait.

Chrysanthia clucked a little over the low-scooped neckline of her gown and generous view of bare shoulders revealed by the drape of diaphanous blue sleeves caught up at graceful intervals by tiny silver clasps.

Thalia knotted a silken silver cord beneath Dia's breasts, leaving the shifting folds of her loose bodice to hang freely. The gown was a multicolored cascade of gossamer blue, rose, and emerald.

Her palla, more for accent than warmth since the weather was balmy and mild, was yards of sheerest fire-blue silk laced through with silver thread.

She added scent of hyacinth, lightly, to her bare throat and in the smooth inner creases of her elbows. Dia whirled in delight, her flesh tingling and rosy from a steaming bath, the feel of fine silk brushing her skin, sensuous and seductive.

Thus Bold Wolf beheld her, a vision, appearing suddenly in the garden. The soft folds of her raiment fell in tiers of color: emerald blending with the grass, above that the deep hue of pink roses; then elegant sky-blue scoops offering tantalizing glimpses of bare shoulders. Her earth-brown hair, shimmering in sunlight, was wreathed in bright flowers.

Her face was radiant. Bold Wolf caught his breath, then smiled his slow, broad smile which curled the corners of his beard and crinkled his eyes.

She noticed his beard was newly trimmed, close and groomed, and she was struck anew at how manly and handsome was Atawulf. Even with his long blond mane hanging free, braided on either side of his face with Winnifreya's distinctive intertwining of beaded leather strands, even with the military boots, open-toed leather laced to the knee below the white trim of the blue tunic he wore, Dia saw not a barbarian in savage regalia, but a warrior, a king, a man—a strong, bold, and noble man, a man of courage and resolve.

They walked together toward their destination, which Atawulf told her was his secret. They strolled along a colonnaded walkway beside a formal garden patterned with paved paths and colorful flowerbeds laid out like a living mosaic, and they laughed as a group of young boys charged down the colonnade, Atawulf's son in their midst, yelling and chasing each other fearlessly between the King of the Goths and the Imperial Princess.

"Oh, we're going to the dining pool," guessed Dia, "below the waterfall!"

Soon they emerged upon the long oblong pool's rounded end. The elegant pool was bordered by slender marble columns and graceful arches and exquisite statues, replicas of the world's most beautiful sculptures. The crystalline water mirrored so perfectly the delicate marble ring of arches and sculpted figures that the reflection seemed part of the architecture, as though the harmonious whole had been envisioned in the original design—and Atawulf suspected that it had.

The sculptured crocodile of natural green marble sunned on its rock in the middle of the pool, and at the far end the long stretch of picturesque water met the hollow rock cave carved into a green hillock. Through it tumbled and dropped and splashed the myriad waterfalls which formed the sheltered little dining nook.

They strolled slowly beside the pool, which was nestled in a narrow valley. The vale's steep grassy slopes were vivid green speckled with a brilliant yellow coat of flowers. Dia laughed when at her approach some of the flowers flew into the air—yellow butterflies, and white, fluttered among the blooms.

The scent of growing things was heady, heavenly. Dia had never felt more alive, more blessed. This day seemed to be creating magic just for them, and she glanced up at Atawulf with the bloom of spring on her cheeks.

"I love this place," she said. "How did you know?"

"Hear that warbler? He told me."

"No, really."

"I didn't know. Your faithful shadow told me."

"Did she now? Have you and Thalia been conspiring behind my back?"

"Unscrupulously."

"That crafty little actress! She never let on."

"I swore her to secrecy."

Dia laughed, her lilting voice as melodious as the bird's. "I shall have a talk with her about where her loyalty lies."

"With you, of course, Princess. She wanted you to be surprised as much as I."

"Oh, this is heavenly, isn't it? I always imagined this is where the gods dined—the old gods, I mean—when they lived; at least, when I was a little girl I believed they once lived and then became sort of . . . fallen, like Lucifer. Their statues stand all around the pool as if they're just about to plunge in for a swim before dinner. Look, there's Artemis and Poseidon, Apollo, Hermes, Athena . . ."

"I've seen Athena," said Atawulf, gazing at the graceful marble goddess holding shield and spear. "The real Athena."

"You couldn't possibly."

"Aye, it was the one on the Acropolis, at Athens. She stands in the Parthenon, a colossal goddess . . . Have you ever seen her?"

"I've never been to Athens."

"To see her, how she stands regally armored, guardian of the city, with that light in her eyes; you could believe there was a wise power within her . . ."

"I could not. She's but a pagan idol, a false goddess, and has no power to be anything at all. Anyway, she isn't there anymore."

"No? Who could move a statue that huge? And why?"

"An Emperor could. My brother Arcadius had it removed and taken to Constantinople. I believe it was burned."

"For God's sake, *why?*"

"Exactly. For God's sake. The Athenians claimed she protected the city from you and Alaric. They began saying you spared the city because of Athena."

Atawulf's dark blue eyes glittered at her strangely. Then he turned a wistful gaze on the eloquently carved image by the pool.

"They were right," he told her softly. "We spared the city because of Athena. She looked like a queen, wise and generous and just, and Alaric said she reminded him of Winn, so we decided to take the tribute they offered us and leave her city unspoiled."

"Oh."

They strolled on in silence awhile, until Dia paused before a statue of a beautiful youth. Even chiseled marble could not disguise the sensuous curve of those lips, the soulful look in those eyes.

"What does this tell you of Hadrian?"

"Antinoüs? It tells me that Hadrian loved boys. At least, this particular boy; he set images of him everywhere."

Dia stared up at the gracefully posed figure of Antinoüs. "It tells me that Hadrian was only human, after all. When Antinoüs died he tried to make him live again. He put his statue here among the gods; he tried to make him a god—by royal decree. Hadrian was a great Emperor, a greatly ordered mind, a genius, but in this"—she shook her head—"in this he was foolish. Hubris and love made him foolish."

"And grief," said Atawulf, gazing past the marble figure. He spoke words low and rough. "I would have built a thousand statues to Alaric if I believed it would bring him back." Now he turned to Dia. "I wonder if it made it any easier for him? Hadrian, I mean. I wonder if it helped fill the . . . hole where someone used to be."

"I don't know. How could it?" Unknowingly Dia fingered her tiny gold locket, and she made an enticingly vulnerable portrait, her hand hovering near her bosom, her face reflectively sad, and sun-shadows off the water playing across her delicate features. Atawulf reached out gently and touched her elbow.

"How did we get so morbid?" He grinned and offered her his arm. "The day's too fine, too perfect to darken it with gloomy thoughts. All this walking about in the sun makes me thirsty. Shall we?"

She smiled up at him and linked her arm into his. "Most delighted, King Atawulf. I am pleased to walk in the company of such a proper gentleman."

"The pleasure is mine, Princess."

She leaned away from him, studying his face with mock scrutiny. "I wonder at this sudden outburst of protocol. I almost believe you're up to something."

"Why, you wound me, Your Royalty."

"Oh, now I know you're up to something. I call you a gentleman and you don't take offense. I accuse you of secret motives and you answer sweetly. Why, Bold Wolf, you'll be spouting poetry next."

"Now you go too far, woman!" growled the Bold Wolf. "You'll wrest no poetry from me!"

Dia laughed, a sound mellow and low, and the two of them wandered to the other end of the pool where the waters splashed in the artificial cave. Coming into the shady grotto from the warm sunshine, they were grateful for the cool atmosphere of waterfalls. In the semicircle of the dining couches, a wine cart waited. Atawulf brandished a silver goblet and lifted the wine pitcher.

Dia whisked the goblet from his hand.

"I'll pour the wine, thank you," she told him. "I remember the last time I let you bring me refreshment."

"So do I." He grinned devilishly.

"You won't be plying me with unwatered wine this time, Bold Wolf; I intend to keep a clear head." In the mixing bowl, sweet wine had been spiced and diluted generously with water, and now a heady fragrance wafted from the heated bowl. Dia diluted it even further, pouring in more water from a pitcher and stirring the mixture with the ladle. She dipped the sweet, minty wine from the bowl, filling two silver goblets embossed with twining grapevines and birds winging to pluck sweet fruit from heavy clusters.

She lifted both goblets and handed one to Atawulf. As he took it from her hand, their fingers brushed, and his lingered upon hers a heartbeat longer than necessary.

"Strong wine," he said ruefully, looking into the pale liquid, "sharpens the appetite and sweetens conversation."

"And muddles the mind. Today my senses are so sharp and pure and awake that to dull them would be . . . sacrilege, and an insult to this glorious afternoon."

"Maybe," he murmured, "I hoped to take advantage of you."

"I'm not surprised. And you may be sure, Atawulf, that a woman is much more gratified if the man taking advantage of her is not drunk in his cups. Then she is certain it is she who captivates him, not the wine."

"Aye, and a woman seduced clear-eyed and sober is all the sweeter."

"Are you planning to seduce me, Atawulf?" she half-teased,

slanting her gaze aside from his and nonchalantly sidling around the circular dinner table.

"Consider this fair warning."

"Fortunate for me, I watered the wine. I wouldn't want to make it too easy for you."

Atawulf bared his teeth. "I expected no less from the daughter of Theodosius."

"Well," Dia said brightly, maliciously, "I'm famished. Shall we dine?"

The moment they settled upon the softly cushioned couches, slaves appeared silently and magically, gliding forward with laden trays. Atawulf had finally become accustomed to these uncanny arrivals, discovering early on that hidden narrow passageways honeycombed the villa exclusively for the use of the slaves; Hadrian had evidently preferred his servants invisible.

Unobtrusively they laid out the purple silk tablecloth and silver dishes, fingerbowls and napkins and silverware. With her fingers Dia daintily plucked up a pickled artichoke heart and popped it into her mouth. Pronouncing it divine, she spooned up deviled eggs smothered in mushroom-and-cream sauce, and dipped a chunk of steaming white bread into a dish of finest olive oil.

Between courses they conversed, flirting with the subject of seduction and love and spring fever. Then arrived the main course: quail, cooked in spices sweet and sharp, served on a bed of onions, turnips, and asparagus, along with pork pastries spiced with cumin, cinnamon, and cloves, then fried in sweet oil and ladled all over with apricot preserves.

"Delicious," said Dia. She nodded to a slave offering to refill her cup, Dipping her fingers in the water bowl, she signaled that she had eaten her fill.

"From the Emperor's own larder," Atawulf agreed heartily, finishing off yet another pork pie and spearing another slice of quail with the sharp handle of his spoon.

"I wonder at this royal repast."

"A feast for an Imperial Princess."

"You never showed so much solicitousness before."

"I never saw you in springtime before."

"You sound like a courting popinjay."

"Why, Princess, you don't like it?"

"I don't believe it."

Bold Wolf lounged on the couch, waving his refilled cup. "Merely my humble attempt to compete with those elegant, trussed-up young noblemen who used to line up at your atrium door, poetry in hand."

Dia laughed, genuinely amused at the picture. "You seem to think my life was a romantic episode, like those silly plays in common theater."

"Wasn't it?"

"And you seem to think I prefer that sort of thing. I should be insulted."

"Are you?"

"Absolutely."

Salted almonds, chestnuts, and walnuts appeared on the table, along with a dessert of cheese rolled in cinnamon and fried in honey and must. The two diners seemed not to notice.

Atawulf gathered his resolve. Now was the time to approach the subject of marriage—and the time to tell her of the proposal he had long since dispatched to her brother.

"Princess, why aren't you married? Or at least betrothed?"

"I beg your pardon?"

"Granted."

"You are prying." She swirled the wine in her cup intently. "I really don't wish to discuss it."

"Now don't climb on your high and mighty dignity. 'Tis a reasonable question. You're twenty-one years old, not a bad eyeful, nor handful, either, of royal blood, and rich as sin, as I hear it."

Dia sat up abruptly on the cushions and plunked her winecup down on the purple tablecloth, deepening the dye with sweet wine.

"Oh, now, there's the real Atawulf at last," she said caustically. "I knew you couldn't keep it up."

"And you don't want me to." He sat up and propped both hands upon his bare knees. "Admit it."

"Admit what?"

"That those perfumed peacocks with their fancy manners are not enough for you, or you would've married one of them. You prefer a man who speaks his mind and doesn't bow and scrape and kiss the soles of your shoes."

"What an extraordinary picture you paint. Am I supposed to be overcome by these sweet words and swoon into your arms? If this is how you set out to seduce a woman, well, let me—"

"You'll know when I start seducing."

"I will, will I? Oh, please, don't bother."

Atawulf chuckled, a deep rumble of self-congratulation that added fuel to Dia's ire.

"If you wanted flowery speeches and worshipful sighs you would've married that poetry boy, that Captain of the Protectors, who probably swooned away when you favored him with a pouty little kiss."

"You don't know what you're talking about, you . . . you rude, barbaric oaf!"

There emitted a squeak of dismay from the servants' passage, which neither of them noticed.

"Then why did you spurn him?" A wicked light gleamed in Atawulf's eyes as a new thought struck him. "Or did he spurn you, Your Royalty? Maybe your noble gentleman wasn't such a gentleman after all."

If he thought to embarrass her or shame her, he was far, far off the mark. Placidia flushed crimson, her eyes flashed green fire, and she came to her feet, furious.

"You have no right to say such things to me! You know nothing about it, Atawulf, and if you knew the truth you would beg my pardon this very moment! I demand that you apologize!"

"The truth."

"Apologize!"

"For *what?*"

"For insinuating that I was taken advantage of and abandoned by the noblest, kindest, most honorable man in the Empire—in the world! Captain Boniface and I were going to be married, despite everyone, *everyone* opposing us."

Now Dia paced the dining alcove, driven by rekindled rage as the memories rose to the fore of her mind like corpses from the grave. "It was *Serena* who ruined it, *Serena* who deliberately destroyed our lives! Oh, she could not bear it, that I might marry someone besides her precious Eucherius. Not that she cared about him either, not that she cared about *anyone* but *Serena!* She only sought to further her own ambitions by wedding her son to the purple—to *me!*"

Atawulf heard her fury, watched her stiff anger in open-mouthed astonishment. This was a new Galla Placidia, and he would not have interrupted this revelation if all the legions of Rome were storming the walls.

"Ah, yes, she pretended to be such a doting, loving cousin, a dedicated guardian to the Emperor's poor orphaned children, but all she wanted, all she *ever* wanted was to breed us like . . . like prize chickens! And when my brother failed to get children by her daughters, she would move heaven and hell to see me married to her son."

Dia halted in her tirade, stood with her back to Atawulf, her small figure framed in the halo of sunlight and blue water, marble arches and green hills.

"He was so good, so honorable, my Boniface, that when she threatened to expose some crime she discovered his grandfather had committed, when she threatened to drag his whole family into court and break them utterly, he had no choice but to do as she demanded." She shuddered, gathering breath to say the words. "He married at her command, a woman she chose. And being an honorable, Christian man, he . . . we . . . don't you see? She made it impossible for us to ever see each other again."

Dia spun to face him, her silhouette rigid and trembling. "And *that* is why I signed the petition authorizing her execution for treason! I wanted revenge, and I wanted her out of my life forever, so I signed it—gladly! She never loved me. She never loved anyone. She used me, just like she used everyone else. She tried to control me, as though I were her property, as though I were but another jewel in her crown of ambitions, a footstool upon which she could step on her way to the throne. And believe me, any grandchildren of hers bred for the purple would simply be new victims in her lust for power."

And now Dia's voice steadied, low and sure and strong, and Atawulf heard in its timbre the daughter of emperors, the blood of conquerors.

"But I would not let her destroy me the way she destroyed everyone else with her insatiable greed. It was too late for Boniface and me, but she was never going to let go, never going to set me free, never going to pull her talons out of my inheritance. So when the people cried for her blood, when Priscus Attalus brought me the Senate's petition, I signed her petty, spiteful, scheming life away.

"And, before God, I'd do it again."

Atawulf came slowly to his feet and walked toward her, his eyes a study in irony.

She held her head high.

"So now you know."

"You're old Theo's daughter, all right." His voice held a note of awe, of discovery.

"And now you also know why I am neither married nor betrothed. I vowed then, there will be no *arranged* marriages for me. When I marry, *if* I marry, it will not be to further anyone's ambitions but my own."

Atawulf considered that this might not be the best moment to mention the proposal he had sent to the Emperor. He began to wonder if there ever would be a right time.

He moved closer to her, close enough to touch her, wanting to touch her.

"Would you not marry for love, Galla Placidia, or would love be barred from this fortress of yours?"

She raised startled eyes to his, then she lowered dark lashes, concealing the depths of her feelings.

"Why, I suppose I would . . . if the match were . . . advantageous."

"No, Dia, a marriage for love must be for love. The advantages don't make a damn difference."

She raised swift eyes to his again, breathless, and she found she was trembling.

"All that matters is here." Now he did touch her, brushed his fingertips across her heart and lingered there. "And here." His burning touch left her to touch his own heart. She felt hers beat wildly.

"Between us," he growled softly, "there is only this."

His fingertips brushed her face, her hair, caressed her cheek, her temple. She felt she would melt inside. Then his golden head bent to her slowly, the deep gaze of his blue eyes penetrating, and she stood scarcely breathing as his lips touched hers softly. The kiss lingered, his beard tickling, and then the kiss deepened and his hands slid down her bare arms, making her shiver all over.

Abandoning herself to this wonderful river of sensation, she answered his lips with hers, and as his strong arms pulled her toward him, she raised her hands to his shoulders, touching him timidly at first through the blue tunic, then more boldly as he pressed her against him, raising her to tiptoes—or did she rise upon her toes in order to twine her arms about his neck?

They forgot everything but each other, the honey-sweet taste of the other, touching, merging, kissing in the amber glow of the evening sun.

Below the chorus of waterfalls, a lone wavering cheer from the dim passage went unheard.

Lost in him, wrapped in him, Dia knew the most exquisite sensual yearning, and every inch of her flesh pressing against his hard body pulsed with heat. She gasped, a swift indrawing of breath, and opened urgent lips to his.

And Atawulf wanted to devour her, drink her, breathe her, this vibrant woman in his arms. When he could bear the need no longer, he suddenly lifted her in his arms and bore her to the nearest couch, laying her upon the soft cushions and bending over her, ominous blue eyes, dark with turmoil, searing into hers.

She reached up to stroke his beard; he caught her hand, kissed her palm, her wrists, the flowery scent of her silky arm, and as he became aware of the quickening of her breathing he knew he should not be doing this. Another moment and he would be unable to stop.

She was his innocent and naive captive, as virgin as untilled earth, and what right had he to plunder her as though she were spoils of a bandit king?

Bold Wolf hesitated, gazed long into waiting eyes alight with anticipation and fear and desire, her full, sensual lips parted, awaiting his descent, and he had never wanted anything in his life so consumingly as he wanted Dia, and he wanted her now, just as she looked this moment, tousled and excited and willing him to take her. He dipped to taste her wine-sweet kiss once more, knowing he would be lost and not caring, heeding only her warm, moist lips full with desire.

Damn Priscus Attalus!

A frantic flurry and flutter had caught his eye from the dim recesses of the passageway. Priscus Attalus was gesturing and miming and making motions suggestive of beheading.

Atawulf reared his head and glared into the shadowy opening.

"What's wrong?" protested Dia, his deliciously ravaging lips having ripped away from hers. "What is it?"

She struggled to sit up, disappointment and relief waging war within her, but the solid barrier of Atawulf's chest kept her from fully rising.

There was much scurrying and scrabbling in the passageway.

Dia felt as if she were waking from a dream, a deep, seductive dream, and waking was making her cross.

"What is so fascinating over there?" She swiveled her head and twisted from beneath him.

A slave bounded into the open, though "bounded" did not quite describe the impression she had—that he had been roundly shoved from the passageway. He blinked wide brown eyes at the couple and fidgeted uncertainly, then did a manful job of improvising. He bowed low, linked his hands before him, and cleared his throat.

"I . . . just . . . will you be needing anything more, mistress?"

Dia, having hastily sat upright and smoothed her dress, shook her head mutely. She felt her hair tumbling down one side of her neck and, reddening, realized what a spectacle she must look. She would be the talk of the slaves tonight, and the worst of it was, they would be right. She had nearly thrown away her modesty and her virtue on a dining couch in full view of the servants and anyone else who cared to take a peek—and in the afternoon! Only courtesans and adulterers indulged in intimate behavior in daylight, though she had to admit the sun had by now discreetly retired and veiled the cove in blue twilight.

Atawulf waved the slave away, who disappeared hastily into the passage. Dia rose to her feet and attempted to straighten the disarray of her hair. Rescuing her fallen palla, Atawulf's contrite voice rumbled in the cavern.

"Dia . . . I apologize. My behavior was not . . ."

"Gentlemanly?" Dia could not help a slight smile. "I am not altogether innocent, Atawulf, since it never occurred to me to object."

"Aye, but I am the one responsible for your . . . safety." Atawulf draped the palla clumsily about her shoulders. "I could never call myself an honorable man if I despoiled a captive under my protection, Princess."

For some reason Placidia suddenly seemed quite put out with him.

"I am not a wilting flower with no will of her own, I assure you, Atawulf. I . . . I had no intention of letting you *despoil* me, as you so vulgarly put it. I . . . I was simply . . . I thought . . . oh, never mind! It doesn't matter!"

"I, for one, Princess, surrendered my head and my wits without a fight. Except for the interruption, I might have done that which we both would regret tomorrow."

She glanced at him swiftly, her expression confounded between alarm and defeat. Oh, how could she feel such turmoil in her heart? And the truth was that her heart was not the only organ in turmoil. She blushed furiously.

"You can't possibly know what I might regret!" She dared not speculate on what she meant by that outburst; quickly she amended it. "You presume too much if you imagine I was completely overcome by your *merest* kiss. Now, if you will excuse me, I . . . it is unseemly to be seen lingering here in the dark like . . . like . . ." She turned and flicked a wrist at the slave silently lighting the torches. "This man will escort me back to my rooms. Goodnight, King Atawulf."

And Atawulf, staring at her retreating back, raised both bushy eyebrows and mouthed indignantly, *"Merest?"* into the dusk for the benefit of the ghostly, motionless gods poised at the edge of the pool.

"You call that courting?"
"I can do without your sarcasm, Priscus."
"You practically had her for dessert."
"Priscus!"
"And you didn't tell her."

"No, I didn't tell her, and you're damn lucky I didn't."

"Lucky?"

"Don't play innocent with me; I know you heard every word. Why didn't you tell me how she felt about being pushed into marriage? Why didn't you tell me about Serena?"

The old statesman shrugged resignedly. "It never seemed relevant. *Everyone* hated Serena."

12

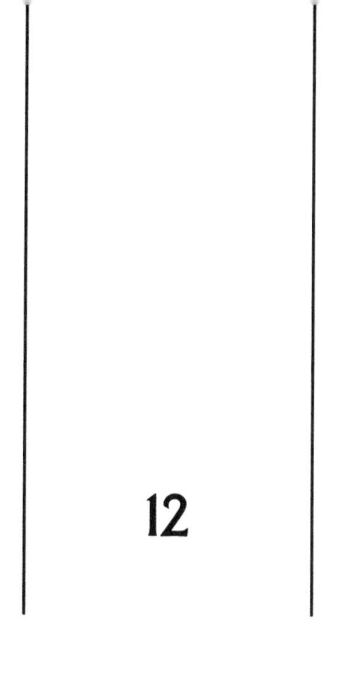

Dia did not return to her apartments. Instead she dismissed the torchbearer and lingered by the gleaming black moat beside the island pavilion. The dark span of the footbridge beckoned her restless feet across the still water. Stars sprinkled the world's black dome, and to the east a silvery aura announced that mistress moon would soon be arriving to reign over the night.

The night was warm, and Dia dropped her flimsy palla on the marble floor and wandered beneath the pavilion, into the palace of columns, pale pillars fading into the deepening shadows.

She leaned her bare back against a cool marble column and stared across the narrow moat into the impenetrable blackness of the garden.

She closed her eyes and relived the moment when Atawulf kissed her. "Would you not marry for love?" he had said with that fire in his eyes, and then he had kissed her.

Love! Yes, Atawulf had spoken the word, and her heart felt it could leap and fly. And she knew now that she wanted nothing in her life but Atawulf. If this pounding, yearning feeling was love, then she loved—from the center of her soul to the tips of her fingers she loved—and if not for that untimely interruption she would have abandoned herself to the wild need within.

If not for the intrusion she would now know the consummation of that terrible, wonderful passion, she would know the heat and strength of Bold Wolf in all his savage arousal, and she would know the mystery, the secret every woman and man in the world must know except Galla Placidia.

Oh, how she regretted that intrusion! True, it had saved her from making a wanton of herself, but at this moment, leaning here against the cool column in the dark pavilion, that was no consolation to her taut body. She felt like a lyre, finely tuned by the musician, and then set aside, no melody played upon her trembling strings.

Would she never know love and all its mysteries? Why could Atawulf not forget that she was his royal captive, his responsibility, and see that she was a woman! If he loved as she loved, ached as she ached, nothing else would matter.

She touched her lips, softly tracing the memory of his kisses. With a longing sigh she turned and wrapped her arms about the column, remembering the feeling of holding Atawulf's powerful body. Cold marble was poor comfort.

Her eyes opened, and she roused from her dreamy imaginings as, in harmonious perfection, music pure and high from a solitary flute heralded the arrival of the moon. Three-quarters full, the night's mistress cast the pavilion in raiment of silver, while vibrant notes from the unseen flute fell through the night like silver rain.

Dia smiled at the beauty of it. The island pavilion transformed into a moon palace, streams of silver light casting stark black shadows across the floor and dancing on the crest of the fountain like stars in the water. The flute's haunting melody seemed to blend with the moonlight, play in the pavilion, call her to follow it; and in the moonlight Dia began to dance.

And Bold Wolf saw her there, his own unspent restiveness leading him to roam the night, and her slender figure bathed in silver light flickered across his vision like a half-glimpsed dream, then disappeared into moonshadow.

He walked on cat feet around the dark moat, wondering if he had imagined her, but she danced back into his vision, bending gracefully to the solemn flute song, her hands weaving the silver air, her hair unbound and flowing, her slippered feet stepping lightly.

The flute tune leapt to a spritely tempo, and the ethereal dancer caught at a slender column and glided around it; she whirled around another and sailed in the moonlight through a white forest of marble, a pagan goddess playing in her temple.

Hidden in a shadowed niche by the wall, Atawulf stood scarcely daring to breathe, and watched the woman in the silvered pavilion, her willowy limbs in supple motion and enchantment upon her uplifted face, soaring on the song of the flute.

The moon and the music wove their magic, and Bold Wolf could stay away from her no longer. He left the alcove and circled the island. A moment later she saw him standing beyond the footbridge, feet planted wide apart, motionless, a sculpted form of masculine beauty washed in silver light.

She stopped in startled surprise, and she might have been marble, poised in the brilliant pavilion as he crossed the footbridge toward her. On he came with his great stride, and her heart stood still. Just a pace away he stopped, the dark pools of his eyes drawing her toward him; she stepped forward but whirled away as his hand reached for hers. She danced a slow circle around him, so close he could have captured her in his arms, and when she moved away, slowly trailing the back of her smooth hand along his corded arm, he did capture her, catching her wrist, drawing her toward him until she pressed against him, heartbeat to heartbeat.

Her eyes invited. He bent to capture her mouth with his, and she let her head fall back, parting her lips to welcome his.

Then they heeded only each other, stirring touch and craving hands, and a heady desire, and they would have devoured each other if they could, so fiercely did they kiss. But Atawulf swept her up and carried her, she freeing one arm and pointing the way to the sleeping nook, and he laid her before him upon the couch.

His touch was like velvet, tender, spreading fire through her flesh, and she, intoxicated with him, senses inflamed, opened her arms to him. Their eyes and lips and hands found each other, and they kissed, savoring, stroking, sighing. His tongue teased her ear as he whispered sweet urgings.

Flame kindled in their flesh, and they shed their garments in a fever.

Then they knew only touch and surging desire, wild raw pleasure and the engulfing fire—fire in their blood, fire in their flesh. And she, the initiate, moaned, yielding to the mystery, the pain, the joy, and they wrestled fiercely, joining, plunging into the flame.

She arched, crying her release, surrendering to the power he unleashed in her, and they yielded to each other, melted, flowed together, panting in unison, sighing, laughing, and tasting the sweat like sacrament.

Entwined, they lay across the couch, Dia cozily resting her head upon his shoulder, both smiling into the night. Later they padded across the silver floor and drank from the moonlit fountain, sipping cold water from one another's cupped hands.

Still later they donned their clothes and, reluctant to part, strolled hand in hand under the moon's luminous gaze, crossing the bridge into the garden. They spoke in whispers, like children creeping adventurously in the shrubbery, until they stole past the balcony and reached the sheltered wall near the vine-cloaked crack. Settling on the silver grass, they leaned together against the wall and stared skyward.

The scent of honeysuckle suffused their bower, and Dia breathed the air ardently.

"Lovely," she sighed.

"Aye."

"And the moon—the most beautiful I've ever seen."

"Aye."

"Did you ever notice? She's like a jewel, gleaming up there in the night."

"Aye."

She turned to look at him. "What are you thinking?"

He smiled. "Shhh. Listen."

She listened. The flute had fallen silent. The night was quiet, still, but the longer she listened to the silence, the more she heard. A chirruping night-bird far in the distance, the invisible chorus of crickets, a gentle wind rattling leaves overhead . . . sounds which only deepened the silence.

She felt a sense of stillness lying over the land, all the world at peace.

"Do you hear?" he whispered.

"The hoot owl?" she whispered back.

"Aye. He's hunting in the moonlight." Atawulf leaned his head back, listening, and she thought he had forgotten her until suddenly he answered her question.

"I'm thinking this is the closest to peace I've ever come. This is what I always imagined peace would be. This night, this quiet, and this place . . . it seems like paradise. I feel I could stay here forever, nothing changing, ever, and be content."

"Me, too."

Bold Wolf's gaze fell on her, his dark eyes catching silver light. *Aye, only if you are here with me.*

"If it were possible . . ." he mused. "I wish my people could settle here."

"Seriously?" She sat up and looked at him.

"I once believed that to be a great chieftain, I must be the best warrior, build the strongest army, and lead my people to victory in war."

"But now?"

"Now I believe the greatest thing a chieftain—or a king—can do for his people is find them peace. I want so much for my people, and they've endured too much wandering, too much war, too much . . . we are a lost people, Dia. We need homes for our children, we need farms and cattle and prosperity, and we need peace. Aye, most of all, peace."

Dia gazed at him, her eyes soft and glistening in the moonlight.

"I hope you find it, Bold Wolf," she said gently. "I hope . . . I wish this enmity would end between Roman and Goth. If only the fighting could be put aside, even for a little while, if your people and my people could live together side by side, each would see how little difference there is between us." She reached up to stroke his face, lovingly. "Just as we have."

He caught her hand, kissed the delicate pulse of her wrist.

"Aye. If they felt as I feel now, there would be naught but love between Goth and Roman."

"We could show them, Bold Wolf." Her eyes glowed with excitement. "We could proclaim our love to all the world, tell them what we know, and call on them to lay down their hatreds and their selfish bigotry. And when they do, when your people and my people learn to meet on common ground, they'll come to know what we know—that we all have the same hurts and needs and dreams, and we all want peace."

And she, being young, believed with all her heart that it could be done, that they need only show the world their discovery, and in the blissful light of love she believed that no one could be so blind as not to see the truth, so hard as not to desire the truth.

He looked into those heaven-sent eyes and could not destroy her innocent trust in human nature. Aye, that would come soon enough, he thought. Too soon.

He had not forgotten the proposal to her brother, the fancy document designed to confound Ravenna, the strategy demanding marriage with Dia to seal the bargain.

Nor did he forget her cousin Serena, and what he had learned this day about Dia's passionate fury.

He should tell her now, he knew, but he dreaded to see the love in those glowing eyes turn to horror and hurt.

"Dia . . ."

Her eyes waited, expectant, trusting.

"Aye," he said, "we'll tell the world, you and I . . ."

He touched her unbound hair and brought away a sprig of honeysuckle. Kissing her lingeringly, trailing his fingers through her hair, caressing her neck, brushing gentle lips down the soft curve of her throat, he knew he was incapable of telling her, not now, not tonight. Slowly, savoringly, they rekindled the fires still smoldering within. They moved together, kneeling, and he drew her silky garment up over her hips flinging the gown aside and baring her to the night.

Her round breasts and smooth belly gleamed in the pale moonlight, and he cupped her radiant skin in warm palms. She shivered, absorbed in the feel of him, searching for him. Heat coursed his veins, phallus silver-lit, he threw off his tunic, and lay her back in the cool grass.

They made love with tantalizing, slow movement, senses arched and quivering, alive in fingertips, lips, and loins in the prickling grass; the sharp smell of sex and sweat mingling with the scent of sweet earth and honeysuckle. Their soft moans and gasps joined the rhythmic cadence of night noises. As one they trembled on the peaks of sensation, panting, arching, and at last embracing the wild plunge into their primeval union.

The universe stilled, stars sharpened against velvet black, a gem-sparkled robe carelessly draped upon the heavens by the naked moon on her way to bed.

Bold Wolf smiled happily, his fingertips tracing lazy spirals around Dia's breast. She sighed, the most luxurious contentment spreading warmly throughout her body. They lay immersed in the moment, and Atawulf saw a streak of fire cross the sky.

"Look! A falling star!"

"Oh, I missed it!"

"There's another—and another! So close I could catch them!"

Dia laughed. "Those are fireflies, silly." She sat up. "Look, the garden is full of them."

He rose to sit beside her, to see the darkness asparkle with tiny golden fiery lights, streaking and fading, an enchanted garden invaded by fairies.

"Oh, they're lovely, aren't they? They come every year. When I was a little girl, I used to chase them and catch them, too. I thought I could capture the pretty lights and keep them in a jar forever." Her voice fell to thoughtful solemnity. "But the fireflies died. They couldn't live in a jar. I remember crying because I killed them and I hadn't meant to. After the first ones died, Thalia and I let the rest of them go."

She paused to watch the sparkling show. "They're not for us to keep. They only shine when they're free."

She looked so solemn, watching the fireflies with childlike intensity, Atawulf wasn't sure whether he wanted to laugh or hug her. So much serious contemplation over a lot of fireflies—he wondered what she was thinking about so deeply that she forgot he was sitting there. But he watched the fairy lights because she did, something he had not done since he was a very small boy.

And if he had known what she was thinking, he would have been surprised, for her own thoughts were surprising her. Memories of her childhood were opening her eyes to something she should have seen all along, and there in the garden she came to a very startling decision, and the idea made her smile as she imagined what she was going to do.

She might have spoken her thoughts aloud to Atawulf if a

commotion had not arisen from the balcony overlooking the garden. They heard Thalia calling, and Rayard, and a clattering down the marble steps.

"Oh, hell, they're looking for us," hissed Atawulf. "Put on your clothes." He flung her dress at her, and hurriedly, laughing under their breaths and fumbling, they slipped on their clothes. Like children caught playing in a forbidden place, they scurried across the garden, and while Atawulf went to confront Rayard, Dia slipped up the steps, giving Thalia a start.

"Oh," said Thalia, seeing Atawulf's departure and her mistress's disheveled appearance. The handmaiden blushed. "I . . . I was worried when you never returned, Miss Dia, so I found Rayard and . . . oh, dear . . . I've blundered, haven't I?"

"No, no, I daresay you've saved me from catching a chill. Let's go in, and I'll tell you all about it."

And by the first glimmer of dawn Dia had indeed told Thalia everything—well, *nearly* everything about the magical evening she spent with Atawulf.

"The most wonderful moment of my life, Thalia. As Dulcie would say, I've been plucked, and I loved every moment. Nothing, nothing can compare. I love Atawulf with all my soul, and I know he loves me. We spoke of declaring our love to the world, which is all but a betrothal. In fact, I'm sure he means to ask me formally, possibly tomorrow, and of course I'll say *yes*."

She awakened with a happy smile and stretched luxuriantly. She was a woman fulfilled now, a woman in love, and the world smiled upon her. She arose to greet the day—nearly midday by now—and discovered she was sore in private places, just as she ought to be, she thought happily.

She sponged off quickly from a basin, for she was ravenous and wanted breakfast. And tearing into a meal of soft bread and honey, figs and almonds and thrice-watered wine, she smiled and hummed and her eyes sparkled with some secret delight when she looked at Thalia.

"Dear, dear, Thalia . . ." began Dia, shaking her head and smiling.

Thalia's black brows rose expressively. So she was "dear" this morning? What had the man done to her mistress?

"I caused you a sleepless night, didn't I? But you needn't have worried; you knew I was with Atawulf. Oh, we made such plans, plans to share our secret with the world. We intend to show everyone how incredibly stupid and tragic is this enmity between Roman and Goth, how far beyond all that warring is our love."

Dia, eager to be fresh and lovely for Atawulf, had Thalia gather things for a real bath, though she hurried and chatted through it, skipping her usual soak in the hot water. Then she fidgeted impatiently while Thalia worked the tangles out of her hair, and her handmaiden commented wryly on the bits of leaves and grass caught on the brush. When Thalia asked which scent she wished to wear today, Dia would have only one.

"Honeysuckle. Honeysuckle every morning. I believe I shall wear nothing but honeysuckle for the rest of my life."

Thalia, behind her, rolled her eyes.

Arrayed in a soft gown of turquoise, her hair plaited singly at the sides and the plaits looped back to adorn the rich brown tresses falling freely about her shoulders, she chose simple mother-of-pearl jewelry to complement her rosy complexion. Then with lively steps she burst upon the peristyle surrounding the grand courtyard—an area empty of horses now but not yet recovered enough from their rough hooves to bear any resemblance to a garden—where she was greeted by bright sunshine and a few familiar faces. For a moment she wondered if they knew what had transpired last night right under their noses, but of course, who would tell them? Certainly not Thalia or Rayard.

She returned their greetings with gracious nods and, Thalia at her heels, continued unhurriedly, she hoped, toward one of the grand atriums, for she could not bear waiting about her apartments all afternoon. Perhaps Atawulf would be about doing kingly business and making kingly decisions, and the atrium seemed a likely meeting place.

Ah, but the atrium was deserted, for what Goth would be indoors on such a day as this? But then she heard muttering in the tablinum. She ascended a few wide steps of black marble and, upon reaching the spacious area, peered around an Imperial-purple curtain into a richly ornamented office.

"Priscus Attalus," she said. "Only you would be at work on such a glorious afternoon."

The speckled bald head, which had been bent in deep concentration over a desk, shot up in alarm. The heavy parchment beneath his startled hands curled up with a snap and bounded to the floor, bouncing and rolling out of her sight.

"Nobilissima!" gasped Priscus Attalus. He staggered to his feet, knocking over the stool he vacated, and looked around the floor wildly before remembering to bow to the Imperial Princess.

"Whatever is the matter with you, Priscus?" laughed Dia, approaching the desk. "You look as if you've been caught in some deep dark conspiracy."

Priscus Attalus managed the remarkable feat of becoming pale and flushed in the same moment, which gave his aged skin a frighteningly mottled look.

"Are you ill?" worried Dia, coming around the desk.

"No! I mean . . . yes, I think I may be quite ill, nobilissima. If you will be so kind as to excuse me . . ."

He snatched up the fallen parchment on which she even now had her eye, and she could not fail to notice that the parchment was Imperial purple with gold-tasseled ties. And did she see the Imperial seal as well? He clutched the wretched parchment before him, in danger of crushing it.

Feeling oddly relieved and miserable at the same time, Priscus was glad this moment had come. He would tell her now, tell her everything, and let Atawulf bark as he would. He took a deep breath.

"Princess Placidia, I have a confession to make. You were not to see this document . . ."

But Dia smiled, thinking she had surprised the statesman in the drafting of a formal marriage proposal, delighted that Atawulf had wasted not a moment of precious time.

"Don't look so guilty, Priscus. I know what it is you are holding."

Priscus gaped. "You do?"

"But of course. Why shouldn't a woman know of her own betrothal?"

Priscus Attalus gave a long sigh of relief. "Then King Atawulf told you."

"Told me? He could scarcely make such a decision without my knowing. May I see? The contents are not secret from the bride-to-be, are they?"

"No-o," Priscus said hesitantly. "I suppose you are entitled . . ." Reluctantly he placed the scrolled parchment in her hand. "I hoped King Atawulf might break this news to you more . . . delicately."

"Oh, he has." She blushed faintly, remembering last night. Priscus, however, merely looked confused, for Atawulf had not yet seen this document and could not know its contents. Dia's eyes scanned the gold-flecked script, the gilding very dry for a fresh draft, and leapt from the salutation at the top to the signature at the bottom.

Her brow furrowed in puzzlement. "Why, this is a missive to Atawulf from the Emperor's Quaestor."

"Yes, it arrived just this morning. I haven't yet had a chance—"

"It's a reply to a proposal Atawulf sent my brother more than a month ago!"

"Well, yes, they took some time to—"

"Just what is this all about?"

"I thought you understood. Didn't the king explain . . . ?"

"Explain? No, he did not!"

"Oh, dear, I fear I've made a terrible—"

"Shut *up,* Priscus, and I will read for myself what you have done!"

And read it she did, every word, the whole sordid story becoming perfectly clear—Atawulf's demand for equal status as a sovereign ruler, a new treaty with the Empire, a proposal for deeded land in exchange for military alliance, and marriage to the Imperial Princess to be the proof of the bargain. The reply, of course, denied each request, point by point. But, oh, there was more, much more. Dia groped to steady herself, sank upon the stool which Thalia righted behind her.

The document not only warned that any marriage between her and the Goth would under no circumstances be recognized by the Emperor, but it scoffed at Atawulf's demand that Galla Placidia's personal inheritance be part and parcel to the alliance.

She felt the shock like a blow to her midriff. For a moment she thought she would never breathe again, then a horrible wrenching twisted in her gut and she wanted to be sick. Gripping the parchment in shaking fingers, she shook her head to clear her suddenly clouded vision.

"He . . . he sued for alliance and my . . . my property?"

"Oh, no," hastened Priscus Attalus, "the property would be yours, of course."

"But he asked for it specifically?"

"Well, yes, but it was all part of—"

"Over a *month* ago? While I was ill?"

"Yes," admitted Priscus shamefacedly. "He never really expected the Emperor to agree to the proposal . . ."

"Then tell me why, Priscus Attalus," Dia said so faintly the old man could scarcely hear her, "tell me why he sent it."

No matter the cost, he would now tell her the truth. "Atawulf felt the proposal would . . . well, he was stalling for time."

"Stalling for time." She repeated the words as though each one

were poison, her own voice hollow in her ears, desolate, disbelieving, yet knowing every word was true. And if that were true, what of last night? What of that charade, that mockery, that *deceit* he had practiced upon her oh, so willing body?

Shame engulfed her, shame and outrage.

"I wanted to tell you, nobilissima; I begged him to tell you immediately, but when he decided he would marry you after all—"

"*He* decided! And when was *I* to be consulted in all this? And where were *you*, Priscus Attalus, all this time? How could you do this to me?" She bit down hard on her lip, fighting back a painful sob. "How could he?"

Mother of God, what a fool she had been! What a simpering, lovesick fool!

She came to her feet, trembling. "Get out of my sight."

"Nobilissima, please."

"*Traitor!* Get out of my sight!"

Priscus Attalus blanched, shaken, but he knew the accusation was real, and no words of his could gloss over the truth of it. Stiffly he bowed and fled the tablinum.

Dia stood, staring trancelike at the swaying curtain, then she sank heavily onto the stool, one gripping sob of anguish ripping through her throat. She dropped her arms upon the desk, cradled her head in them, and, fists clenched, fought the rising tears.

Very softly Thalia stepped forward and laid a gentle arm across her shoulders, but she knew no words to soften this grief. But her touch roused Dia, for Dia was not yet ready to succumb to tears. Tears were for scorned maidens; wrath was for the daughter of Theodosius.

Sitting impatiently erect, Dia spread the hideous purple document on the desk before her, moving it better into the light streaming from one high window. She spread her fingers across the crinkled parchment and began reading.

"Don't read it again, Miss Dia," said Thalia. "Don't."

"I want to be certain I understand every word, every particular." Her voice was ragged, but determined. Yet, determined as she was, the gold script rippled and blurred and finally disappeared altogether as her eyes welled with unbidden tears. She blinked, refusing them release.

That was when Priscus Attalus returned with Atawulf, frantically ushering the Gothic king into the tablinum, having spewed the whole garbled story out at him, along with a few recriminations of his own.

She looked up, and the eyes that met Atawulf's were oceans of pain, and his heart wrenched, for he knew he was the cause of that pain. But shards of ice glittered behind that pain.

As she watched Atawulf approach, she searched for the monster, the unfeeling schemer whose ambitions had stolen her innocence, but his eyes met hers steadily, clear lapis-blue, and his brow was furrowed—with what, worry? Ah, he might well be worried, she thought searingly. All his ambitious schemes gone awry.

He came right up to the desk, glancing down only once to take in the purple parchment beneath her hands, then his eyes returned to hers, searching, and he leaned forward and laid his broad hands over her clenched fists.

"Dia . . ."

She jerked her hands away as though he were poisonous, leapt to her feet, the desk between them.

"Have you no shame?" she spat at him.

"Dia, listen to me . . ."

"Oh, why, so you can tell me lies? Tell me this is all a misunderstanding?"

"It isn't what you believe. I love you . . ."

"Don't . . . don't say that to me."

His gaze met hers with an intensity that fairly crackled in the air. Hers crackled back, seastorm meeting thunderstorm. He shook his head.

"I won't."

"Good, because I won't believe it."

"What will you believe?"

"Nothing you say. You've been lying to me—"

"No."

"Deceiving me, then. You sent this proposal of marriage to my brother over a month ago. A month! And all this time you've never said a word."

"I should have."

"But you are no fool, are you, Atawulf? You *knew* how I would feel about it . . ."

"How could I?"

"So you . . . you *tricked* me into believing you loved me, when all along it was my property and my usefulness in making bargains with my brother!"

Atawulf's jaw clenched and dark flame flickered in the depths of his eyes. His words were low and strained.

"Do you truly believe that, Dia?"

"How could I not?" She raked up the crackling parchment and shook it at him. "I am not merchandise to be bargained like tradesgoods!" She took a heaving breath, steadied herself, leaned a hand upon the desktop. "What I don't understand, Atawulf, is how you expected me never to find out. You couldn't keep it from me indefinitely. And you must have known my brother would never agree to such an abominable match."

Atawulf looked as if he had been struck an unexpected blow. His words grated roughly.

"It wasn't so abominable last night."

"How dare you throw last night at me! *I* at least was *sincere!* What was it to you?" Suddenly she half laughed, a high, thin sound of anguish from the verge of hysteria. The next words were the hardest she had ever said, but say them she would because to veer away from the ugly truth was to confirm what he had thought of her.

"Oh, I see clearly now. It was so simple, wasn't it? So easy?" The words caught on a sob in her throat. She swallowed it back and retreated into fury. "You decided to convince the gullible, naive little fool that you loved her, and she'd be so smitten she'd believe anything you said. And then, to be *sure* . . . oh, God . . ."

Shaking, she pressed one hand over her eyes. She looked so hurt, so wounded, that even now Atawulf started around the desk toward her, but she shrank from his touch and jerked away, so that the stool stood between them.

"Is that why you made love to me?" She shuddered, her voice a barely audible whisper. "To consummate your precious alliance? In case my brother wouldn't recognize a union? Or to be sure I would be . . . *spoiled goods* and have to marry you anyway?"

Now Atawulf's voice turned nasty. "You couldn't be wrong, could you?"

She looked into his eyes and saw bitter anger. God in Heaven, she wanted to be wrong, but the damning proof was right here, clenched in her fist. She flung the document in his face and whirled away from him, rounding the desk and fleeing across the room.

Thalia followed, her jet-black eyes on Atawulf, full of sad accusation.

Dia passed the ashen-faced Priscus Attalus without a glance, but when she reached the purple curtain she stopped, biting her lip and blinking toward the ceiling, struggling for dignity, for control. She spun to face Atawulf's glowering form, her eyes glacial, her voice resonant with all the contempt at her command.

"By the way, Atawulf, you could never have gained control over my property. A married woman is not her husband's chattel. Her property is her own. That has been Roman law for hundreds of years. *We* are not barbarians."

She slapped aside the curtain and walked from the room, leaving it ringing with her disgust.

Atawulf stared at the empty space between the curtains, his eyes glittering. He did not deserve that. He never wanted her damned property. He never wanted anything from her except . . . what had he wanted? More than one night in a garden. More than a political arrangement.

He wanted Dia, the beautiful, vibrant woman with the quick

mind and sharp tongue, the soft eyes with love glowing for him, the sensual lover and the haughty princess and the vulnerable woman, even the wrathful fury who had just raked him with her contempt. With her anguish.

He retrieved the parchment and stared at its contents blindly, and part of him wanted to blame the Emperor for sending the damning document. Another part of him wanted to blame Dia for becoming wildly irrational over the merest hint of marriage for alliance. But most of him suffered because he had indeed done this behind her back and kept it from her. Had he not courted her in false skin, a cloak of deceit? Had he not withheld the truth from her for his own advantage in the capturing of her heart?

Atawulf groaned and let the parchment fall and roll up on the desk. He dropped onto the stool and propped his head in his hands, kneading his knuckles viciously into his brow.

What could he possibly do to heal this terrible wound between them? How could he convince Dia of the only truth that mattered—that he loved her?

"Your Majesty?"

"Aye, go on, say it, Priscus. You warned me."

"No, I . . . I'm sorry, Atawulf, just . . . sorry."

Only after she reached her apartments, only after she had managed the long walk, rigid and trembling, head held high, only in the private sanctum of her bedroom, only then did she allow the tattered shreds of her dignity to fall.

She sat on the bed, shaking, squeezing her fingers together, swallowing hard.

She wanted to scream, to tear her throat out with agonizing, wounded shrieking. She wanted to beat her fists raw against something hard and hurtful.

Mother in Heaven, how he had tricked her! He took her love, her body, her virginity with calculated callousness, to ensnare her in his plans, to ensure her cooperation in going through with the marriage.

She felt humiliated, degraded.

She wanted to be angry, not sorry, but her anger was swallowed up in an overwhelming flood of grief.

She sat on the bed, hot tears overflowing, racked with sobs, and Thalia sat beside her and held her, rocked her, and shed a few tears herself for her mistress and friend. Hours, it seemed, she cried, for every time she tried to overcome the choking, painful weeping, a new bout of shuddering overwhelmed her. Crying was agony, but at least it was endurable agony. The loss and betrayal were not.

At last she huddled on her bed, having cried until her eyes ached, her throat hurt, her every emotion exhausted and raw.

Thalia brought her honeyed wine and gently coaxed her to drink. Dia sat on the bed, gripping the cup and trying to swallow past the knot of grief in her throat.

"I feel like a weepy little girl," she confessed shakily.

"If it makes you feel better . . ."

"No, it doesn't make me feel better—nothing's going to make me feel better. Oh, Thalia, I thought . . . I really believed he . . ." She choked on the word *loved,* unable to voice the unendurable.

That was the worst of it—she had believed their love was genuine, pure, as though blessed by Heaven and smiled upon by angels, nothing sordid or worldly about it. But not so for *him!* He had wanted her only for her market value in a bid for alliance and land.

"All along I was just some . . . game piece he maneuvered this way and that, thinking he could use me to get what he wanted from my brother. I feel so stupid!"

She swallowed a mouthful of wine noisily.

Nothing ever changed. People only cared about her for her proximity to the purple, for the ambitions she could fulfill. Oh, yes, she was feeling utterly unwanted and unloved.

She laughed, a harsh, bitter sound. "Well, Atawulf miscalculated. He didn't get a single concession from my brother. No alliance, no land, no ransom." She sobbed into the winecup.

Thalia passed her a fresh linen handkerchief. "Perhaps those were not Atawulf's only reasons. Miss Dia, he tried to explain—he tried to tell you he loved you."

"Thalia, how could he? He . . . *used* me. Well, if he imagines that what he did to me last night will make a difference, that I'll be forced to wed him anyway . . ." Dia stared into space, stumbling upon a new misery. "Oh, Holy Mother, what if . . . what if I'm pregnant?"

"You could find out. I'll fetch Chrysanthia; I've heard her say there are times you're more likely to get pregnant than not. I'm sure she'll know."

"Don't you dare. I'm so humiliated. I feel so degraded." Dia bubbled into the handkerchief and wiped her nose. "You can't imagine what it feels like to be treated like a piece of . . . *merchandise.*"

Thalia sat back on her heels and regarded the princess with lustrous, solemn eyes.

"Oh, I can, Mistress Dia," the handmaiden said softly.

Dia glanced up, astonishment in her eyes. The next moment she looked contrite, ashamed.

"Of course you can, Thalia. If I were myself, I never would have said such a thing. You know that, don't you?"

"I know, miss."

Momentarily forgetting her misery, Dia studied Thalia's quiet, narrow face.

"Do you sometimes wish you were free, Thalia?"

The midnight eyes widened, then the fringe of black lashes lowered over them. "Everyone does sometimes, miss."

"When do you think about it?"

Thalia looked at her locked fingers, clearly uncomfortable with the conversation. "I . . . I thought about it most when Dulcie was . . . when the Goths made her one of them. I . . . wondered how it felt. That's all."

And at the mention of Dulcie, the next question on Dia's mind went unasked. She was going to ask, *What would you do if you were free?* but the abrupt reminder of what Dulcie had done stopped her. Dulcie had simply left Dia, abandoned her, and Dia could not contemplate another loss—especially not Thalia—and she didn't think she could bear Thalia's answer.

Without warning, new tears spilled from the corners of her eyes, trickling hot and wet into the winecup.

"Honorius never offered ransom for me, just as though he never cared one bit that I was in the hands of barbarians who might do God-knows-what to me."

Thalia dipped the handkerchief into the water basin and wrung the dripping cloth. She dabbed soothingly at Dia's chafed face with the cool dampness.

"Plenty of people love you, Miss Dia," Thalia told her earnestly.

"Who?" puckered Dia miserably.

Thalia's words were softly spoken, but undaunted. "I do, for one, miss, and maybe I know you better than anyone."

Dia smiled then and blinked moist, reddened eyes at her handmaiden. "Oh, my sweet Thalia, you know just what I need to hear. Don't think I don't appreciate you, because I do."

Thalia braced herself for what she had to say next, words she had saved until Dia might be ready to hear them.

"Despite everything, miss, even despite what he did, I think Atawulf truly loves you, too."

The explosive outrage Thalia half-expected did not come. Instead, Dia's eyes welled with pain.

"Oh, Thalia," came her barely audible whisper, laced with regret, "I wish I could believe it. I wish I could believe it were true."

• • •

Atawulf could not shake the look on Dia's face from his memory. That haunted, wounded look of betrayal. Aye, if he could go back a month, he would do it all differently. Why had he not seen what finding out this way would do to her? He should never have kept it from her, he should have laid his plans before her immediately and not hidden them like a guilty secret while every day he fell deeper and deeper in love with her. Knowing she would be hurt.

But he hadn't known how deep the knowledge would cut until it was too late. He hadn't known of the festering wounds she already suffered over being used for political expediency. He hadn't known how mortal a blow this would be to her trust. And her love.

Cursing his stupidity, he paced the top level of the double-tiered colonnade overlooking the swimming pool and park. Cursing himself—and her.

Remembering the icy contempt in those sea-storm eyes, he struck the balustrade with his fist, but the biting pain in his knuckles was no match for the pain in his heart.

Why had she been so quick to believe he never loved her? So quick to believe he was naught but a cruel and calculating predator?

Bold Wolf's heart had opened to her as it had to no other woman, and she called him liar and deceiver. What meant the night of complete surrender to each other in the garden? How could she believe that had been no more than the machinations of ambition, of callous greed?

His throat clenched in pain. Atawulf leaned on his palms against the balustrade and stared northward, away from the villa, toward the lush green trees sweeping wispy clouds across an azure sky, but he saw only his own black turmoil.

Had his touch, his love, said no more to her than that?

God, he hurt in a way that turned his guts inside out.

Aware of movement at the end of the colonnade, Atawulf turned his head to see a familiar figure approaching through the slanted shadows. Wallia.

Atawulf looked back toward the horizon, then bowed his head and pressed at the corners of his eyes with thumb and forefinger. With a resolute breath he stood erect and leaned against a column, awaiting his brother.

Wallia joined him, resting against the nearest column, crossing his boots at the ankles.

"Woman trouble, brother?"

"Aye. You're a good guesser, Wallia."

"I wrung it out of the old man. I'm not blind, you know. One minute you're sheep-eyed in love, the next you're a snarling wolf. Don't take it so hard; she'll get over it."

Atawulf shook his head. "She believes the worst of me. I tried to tell her . . . she would hear nothing I had to say."

"They never do when they think they've been trifled with. Want a bit of advice from me, big brother?"

"You?" Atawulf grinned slightly. "What do you know about women, youngster?"

"More than you."

"All right, tell me."

"Women live in their emotions, and their emotions are like the weather. One day stormy and all tears, the next day balmy, all sunshine and smiles. *Reasoning* with them in the midst of a tempest is . . . well, do you reason with a rainstorm?" Wallia shook his head, the man of experience reproving youthful folly. "You take cover until it blows over. Same with women."

Atawulf swallowed hard against the knot in his throat. He glared across the rolling horizon.

"Are you saying a woman's love is as inconstant as the weather?"

Wallia frowned, his analogy turned against him. "No, not her love; if she loves, she's constant. But her emotions are another matter."

"So what's your advice, brother?"

"Give her a couple of days. Hell, give *yourself* a couple of days; you're no pillar of Hercules yourself. Two days and she'll have calmed down, thought better of it, and be ready to forgive anything."

"Forgive," muttered Atawulf savagely. "I don't want forgiveness! I want to know why she'd rather believe my love was a lie than listen to what I have to say!"

"Aye. If she loves you, she'll listen." Wallia clapped him heartily on the shoulder. "Two days. I promise. Come on, Bold Wolf, saddle that red beast of yours and we'll stretch our horses' legs. The ride'll clear your head."

"Maybe you're right. Maybe in two days I won't give a damn whether she listens or not."

Wallia shook his head and grinned crookedly. "Now you're talking like my hard-headed brother."

Two days and he had not come. Two days and Dia had closed the curtains and turned away all visitors, even Priscus Attalus . . . *especially* Priscus Attalus, traitor.

Two days and Atawulf had not come.

Holy Mother, how she wished he would come to her and say it was all a misunderstanding, convince her that he loved her and that nothing else mattered.

But would she believe him if he did? She didn't know.

She only knew he had not bothered himself about her. All the more evidence that she meant less to him than the possibility of treaty with the Empire.

Well, the daughter of Theodosius certainly was not going to go crawling to a barbarian and make a fool of herself.

Two days. She had to face the truth. He did not love her after all. She kept the curtains closed because she couldn't bear to see the sunny skies or hear the birds trilling or smell the honeysuckle. She stayed in and moped, and drove Thalia to distraction.

Two days. Atawulf admitted to himself that he had needed those days to clear his mind. His initial guilt and anger and hurt had balled into a cold, hard resentment that weighed like a stone in his heart.

The King of the Goths would not go crawling to some spitting Roman cat. There seemed nothing to say. If he told her he loved her, would she believe him? He was not ready to face the possibility that she might turn eyes full of cold contempt on him and call him a liar.

Two days. Atawulf avoided the grand peristyles and brooded on his lack of courage.

"Young man, if you can stop gaping long enough to call off your ruffians, I suggest you inform your king—whatever-is-his-name?—that Imperial Princesses Justa and Grata demand to see their niece."

The Goth on the wall realized he was indeed gaping and snapped his mouth shut. He stared at the occupants of the carriage in amazement. Two women, with only two attendants and a handful of armed guards—*dis*armed by now and looking nervous—had trotted boldly up to the villa to come calling.

"Well?" demanded the thin one, her head thrust out the carriage window, her dark hair limp and dusty. She did not look like his notion of an Imperial Princess, but then again, he had seen Princess Placidia in such a travel-worn state.

The other one, the plump one, lifted her netted veil and looked out the other window.

"Are you or are you not in charge here?"

"Aye . . . ma'am."

"Now we are getting somewhere," said the thin one. "Kindly open this gate and inform your king . . ."

"Justa, I do believe he thinks we're spies."

"Nonsense. Spies do not declare themselves at the gate. Young man, we are here about the *ransom* of Imperial Princess Galla Placidia. Just tell your King Wolf that."

"Oh, aye, King Wolf will want to hear about that. Open up; let 'em through."

"There, Grata, I knew mention of ransom would do the trick. You see, we've embarrassed him."

"I don't know. I think he's laughing."

The guard, ducking his head, was attempting to conceal a broad grin. Lord, two more of them. He sent a runner right away to inform "King Wolf" he had royal visitors.

King Wolf would have guessed they were of the royal family even if Dia had not spoken of her aunts many times in connection with her childhood visits to the villa. Though the women had to be in their early forties, both had a youthful appearance. Justa's sparse flesh was creased more from wind and sun than time, while Grata's pink round face revealed almost no trace of age at all. The family resemblance showed in their eyes, in the shapes of their mouths, and in the graceful gestures of their hands, and that imperious inflection in their voices.

Born and bred Imperials. Atawulf grinned.

"Welcome, ladies, Princesses, Your Royalties."

"King Wolf," acknowledged Justa, with a bare raising of her brows. "We are here to see our niece."

"A social call?"

"We intend to ascertain that she is unharmed and to arrange for her release."

"Ah, and you've brought ransom?" Atawulf eyed the carriage skeptically.

"Certainly not. We're not fools. However, arrangements can be made."

"After we've seen her," added Grata.

"Are you from the Emperor, by chance?" Atawulf prodded cautiously.

The sisters glanced at each other, long-standing scorn for the present Emperor flashing between them.

"We are not!" declared Justa. "We have resources of our

own; we do not need Honorius. *If* you indeed have Princess Placidia—and you must take us to her at once to prove it—we will discuss terms."

"She is here, isn't she?" broke in Grata pleadingly. "We must see her. We've come such a long way."

"Grata, don't beg."

Grata hissed under her breath at her sister. "Men love a woman in distress, Justa. You never did understand that."

Atawulf regarded them with what he hoped was a forbidding glower. "Aye, she's here." He snapped his head around to the runner. "Inform Princess Placidia that her aunts are here to see her. I'll be bringing them up."

As Hadrian had not designed his villa for carriages, Atawulf escorted the royal sisters on foot.

He looked with amusement at their travel-stained clothes; they had made no attempt to conceal their rank or wealth, obviously counting on their identities to afford them protection. The rich, colorful garments hung limp with dust and sweat. A sudden thought stopped him.

"I have riders out. You ladies are lucky you made it here."

"We know all the roads to the villa," Justa informed him. "Even the narrowest wagon track."

Sigeric and his men were out, thought Atawulf. If that band had run across them, the fact that they were royalty would not have saved them from rape and robbery, or death. Even if Sigeric stopped long enough to listen to their story, Atawulf doubted it would have made much difference.

"Foolish," muttered Atawulf. "If you knew how dangerous it was . . ."

"We know the dangers," Justa said curtly. "We've seen the work of your *riders*."

Scarcely believing the news, Dia found them on the plaza and came running, eyes shining. Right behind Dia ran Thalia, and far in the rear puffed old Chrysanthia. There was a great deal of hugging and greeting, weeping and smiling, and the women crossed the plaza arm in arm, Dia tucked between her aunts, chattering like magpies in a cherry tree. As though it were any summer at the villa and they were not in the midst of an invading army.

Women, thought Atawulf. Like the weather.

In the midst of their reunion, Dia was exquisitely aware of Atawulf's close presence, but beyond one seeking glance she pretended he was not there. She was not going to let the anger and confusion she felt when she looked at him cloud her joy in her aunts' arrival. Her eyes misted as she hugged them.

"Oh, you darlings. I can't believe it. You know you shouldn't have. Didn't you know the danger?"

Justa chortled. "My dear, we can tell you about danger! But never mind us . . ."

"How are *you*, Dia?" blurted Grata. "They're treating you decently, aren't they?"

"Yes, oh yes. I'm fine, Aunties." She smiled from one to the other. "Really, and I'm so glad to see you. Thank you for coming. It must have been frightening, the journey, I mean."

Justa shook her head. "Devastating, dearest, just devastating. So many hungry people, so many homes burned. We'll tell you all about it, of course, and you must tell us all about your journey, and about the Goths . . ."

And they chattered all the way to the Imperial apartments. "Why is it so dark in here?" exclaimed Justa. "Open these curtains." A chambermaid scurried to flood the room with light, Chrysanthia saw that refreshments were served in the sitting room, and slaves filled water basins so the women could wash off the road dust. They cooled their thirst with wine and nibbled on cheese and bread and fruit and talked their hearts out.

Dia described some of her journey with the Goths, and her two aunts listened, fascinated, and shaking their heads sadly over the tale of Dulcie's death.

"Of course, our adventures aren't a candle to yours," Grata told her, "but we were raided by Goths."

"We had to flee our estates," said Justa. "We left with practically nothing but the clothes on our backs and rode straight through to Florentia."

"We lived there a month before we worked up the courage to check on our estates. Mine were razed, the orchards and fields and grain houses, and my villa was burned. A blackened hull. Charcoal."

"Oh, no, your beautiful villa!" sighed Dia. "What about yours, Aunt Justa?"

"Not a scratch. They crisscrossed the country rather haphazardly, and they missed mine completely. Grata will have to live with me for awhile."

"I will not," Grata said. "I told you, you are simply too particular. We could never live together."

Dia broke in, "What about your architect? Acasius must've felt awful, all his work destroyed."

"I only wish he'd been there to see it," said Aunt Grata. Her round face puckered in self-pity. "My dear, I've been deserted. The fickle man ran off with an actress."

"Don't exaggerate," Justa told her. "You paid her to seduce him to see if he'd fall for it. You can't blame anyone but yourself if it worked."

"Well, I had to do something. I'm too old to live with a temperamental artist who suddenly decides to fly into a tizzy at every little thing that doesn't go his way. I told him he could just take his fancy girl and his petulance elsewhere. Give me harmony. Let me enjoy my prime years."

Later in the evening, before they retired, Grata took her niece's hand and gazed at her searchingly. "You're unhappy, Dia, I can see it."

"No, Aunt Grata, I'm not. I'm thrilled you're here and I'm so grateful you came through all that danger just to see me."

"But you're sad, too, my girl. Homesick?"

Dia swallowed hard and nodded. "I was beginning to feel no one cared what happened to me."

"Oh, my dear child, we've been frantic. When we heard that the Goths were encamped at the villa, Justa and I came as quickly as we could. Dia, you're our baby, our love."

"I love you, Aunt Grata," Dia whispered, hugging her aunt tight, but she was near tears.

"So what's wrong, sweetie? Have these barbarians been cruel to you?"

"No-o," she sobbed. Then the whole story poured out of her, her love for Atawulf and the plans he had kept secret from her, plans to use her for reasons of his own. Grata and Justa listened and pried and consoled, until, hiccupping, Dia ended with, "I want to go home, that's all, but I don't even know where home is!"

"Your home is with us," Justa said emphatically. "You let us deal with this ruffian king, and just see if he doesn't let you go."

"Since that chicken-breeder of an Emperor won't come up with any ransom, we're prepared to make an offer of our own."

"Grata! Shush!"

"Oh, you wonderful dears. But you just heard what sort of ransom Atawulf was looking for—land and marriage into the Imperial line, not to mention all my inherited properties. You can't offer him enough."

"Just the same . . ."

"He has no reason to hold you . . ."

Dia shook her head wearily, having mulled it over until her brain hurt. "It's true, I believe you're right; he has no more use for me now. He knows he won't profit . . . if that's what he wanted." She had to swallow more tears. "I shall be the one to petition. I'm not afraid to confront him, and I certainly won't allow him to think I'm so humiliated I need to send my aunts in my place.

"Tomorrow. Tomorrow I'll petition him to send me home. If he has any honor, he'll not refuse."

Atawulf agreed to meet Dia in the tablinum immediately upon receiving her message. She wanted neutral ground, and the Emperor's office seemed the appropriate place. The King of the Goths paced restlessly awaiting her arrival; he could guess what she wanted, and he didn't know what his answer would be.

For the tenth time he glanced toward the purple-curtained entryway, and at last there she stood, poised and perfect in the soft light. His heart wrung itself a little tighter, and his mouth went dry as he waved her into the room.

She dipped her head imperiously. Aye, he thought, the aunties have already been at work on her. Hers was the face of royal gravity, still and remote. Well, the King of the Goths could play at masks, too. Atawulf retreated into polite restraint.

She seated herself in a chair before the polished desk. This was harder than she imagined and she found it easier to maintain her poise while seated, easier to disguise the white-knuckled grip beneath her palla and the trembling of her knees.

"I want to know what you intend to do with me."

"What makes you think I have intentions?"

"You must have plans. What are they?"

In fact, he did not. He had distinctly avoided facing that question. He shifted uncomfortably on the stool behind the desk. It was too low for him.

"Since when is the captor obliged to explain his plans to the hostage?"

"Hostage? Now I am a hostage again?" She laughed bitterly. "The marriage ploy was a failure, so we drop the masks and return to the vulgar truth. All right. The truth is my presence here is useless to you. Give up, Atawulf; there is no profit in holding me. The Emperor not only rejects your proposal for marriage, but he will not concede one thing for my release. My God, you can't even make a decent ransom on me! What reason can you possibly have to keep me prisoner?"

Her eyes sought his. Oh, she wanted to hear a reason, one reason—that he couldn't bear to live without her, that he loved her—but his eyes darkened, revealing nothing.

"Prisoner?" he growled. A wave of his hand indicated the

villa around them, implied what he thought of her complaint. "Is your prison too . . . barbaric, Your Royalty?"

She took a steadying breath. "No . . . it is a beautiful, luxurious prison, but I wish to go free . . . I've been kept from my people and my family . . ."

Atawulf snorted. He abandoned the stool and paced around the table. "Does that include your half-brother?"

"I don't see what business it is of—"

"Do you think you'll be better off with the Emperor?" Atawulf ran a hand through his hair, agitated. He didn't want to lose her to that other world, and he could feel her slipping away from him. "Obviously your brother holds the reins on all of your affairs, even your inheritance. A brother who doesn't want his half-sister back in the first place. A brother who probably hoped all along we would conveniently dispose of you."

Dia was on her feet by now, partly because she wanted to hear no more of this, partly because the man towering over her made her feel at a disadvantage.

"Honorius never hoped any such thing! And surely you don't expect him to release my properties knowing a barbarian *bandit* might make use of them."

"I'd bet a year's salt he *never* plans to release your properties."

Fury raged in her aquamarine eyes. Fury because she feared what he said was true, and fury because of what he didn't say, didn't feel. Fists clenched, she drew on that fury to engulf her pain.

"Answer me, Atawulf. Will you release me or no?"

"No." He felt a perverse pleasure in that one word.

She did not ask why. Atawulf wished she had, but would he have answered truthfully? *I love you; I can't give you up!* But she didn't ask. Trembling with barely controlled emotion, she spun around, whipped the curtain aside, and left it swinging in her wake.

13

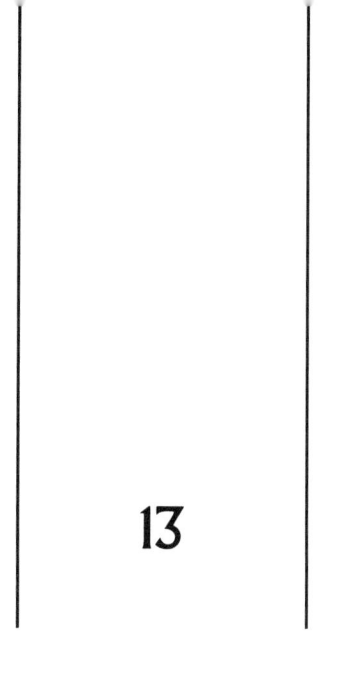

"He refused to even discuss it with me," complained Aunt Justa, having had her turn at dealing with Atawulf.

"You should have let me go instead," Aunt Grata insisted. "I know how to appeal to a man's heart."

"The man hasn't any heart," Dia said sharply. "At least not when it comes to me."

"There now, dear," crooned Grata, "you're not digging deep enough. You know, a few judiciously shed tears wouldn't do any harm."

"You mean grovel?" Justa was appalled. "She'll do no such thing."

"No, absolutely not," agreed Dia, nevertheless feeling a furtive tear luking in her eye. She turned her face to the sun and pretended to sweep back a strand of her immaculately braided hair. She smeared away the offending tear.

"So we find another way," said Justa, undaunted. The three Imperial Princesses with handmaidens and attendants were strolling through the little garden toward the covered portico.

"I *am* excited," admitted Grata. "Barbarian royalty, right here in our villa, and our guests for dinner."

"It's meeting the royal *women* that interests me," Justa said. "I always say if you want anything done, go to the women in charge. You can always reason with a woman."

Their arrival beneath the portico caused a silent stir among the serving slaves. Tables and wicker chairs had been arranged to take advantage of the afternoon shade, and slaves were laying out cushions and tablecloths, fingerbowls, and silverware.

Singledia the Elder arrived, with Winnifreya and her two daughters. The Gothic entourage met the Roman princesses with studied courtesy, and introductions were polite and reserved.

"We're dining in chairs today," Aunt Grata chatted merrily, determined to put the guests at ease. "I understand you prefer chairs over couches, and you're quite right to do so; chairs are much cozier. And I do believe that since women began reclining with men at dinner, our digestion has never been the same."

Dia cut her eyes aslant at Singledia the Elder, wondering what the mother of warriors and kings would make of her aunt's silly prattle, but she need not have worried. A smile played briefly around the older woman's mouth before she puckered her lips and commented in her rich, throaty rasp.

"Gothic women are of the opinion that chairs are for conversation, and couches are for making love."

The daughters of Winnifreya giggled, and Dia blushed, remembering the couch in the island pavilion, but Grata was delighted.

"Oh, a woman after my own heart. Do sit by me; my sister is such a fuddy-duddy. Sit where you like, ladies. Protocol is dismissed for the afternoon."

The women and girls chose seats arranged around two circular tables set close together. As they sank into the plush cushions, slaves placed fragrant garlands of fresh flowers upon their brows.

Dia glanced at Thalia, who stood silently at her elbow, ready to serve anything from the table that her mistress might not conveniently reach.

Justa, who had been counting, looked puzzled. "There are eight chairs and garlands here, and eight places set. I'm certain we told Chrysanthia seven."

Grata counted and shrugged. "She made a mistake."

Dia laughed, unable to withhold her delight. "No, Chrysanthia made no mistake, Aunties. I asked her to set the extra place. We're going to have another guest."

Dia turned and addressed her handmaiden softly. "Thalia, will you join us for dinner?" She gestured toward the vacant seat.

"Miss?" whispered Thalia, startled.

"You are the expected guest." There was no mistaking Dia's intent as she bestowed upon her handmaiden an irrepressible smile, an excited glow in her eyes.

Thalia stood speechless, the black depths of her eyes widening, glistening, staring into Dia's. Thalia knew well the one reason a mistress would invite her slave to sit at table with guests.

"Come and sit, Thalia," Dia said more gently, seeing her handmaiden was too amazed to move. She patted the curved chair. "I saved you the place beside me."

At last Thalia was able to make her stunned limbs move and she came around the chair, not to sit, but to kneel at Dia's feet.

"Miss Dia," she breathed in a rush, gazing up at her seated mistress. "I . . . oh, *thank you.*"

Dia smiled. "No thanks are necessary. You deserve it, and you know you do." Dia lifted the garland of flowers from the empty chair and placed it upon the glossy black crown of Thalia's head. As she settled it into place, she winked at her former handmaiden.

Overwhelmed, Thalia bowed her head upon Dia's knees.

Laughing, Dia caught her hands and stood, raising Thalia to stand beside her. Clasping the trembling fingers tightly, Dia gazed straight into the lustrous dark eyes.

"I declare you a slave no longer, Thalia. From this moment forward, you are a free woman."

Thalia's fingers curled around Dia's. "Oh, Mistress Dia . . ."

"Oh, no, you have earned the right never to call me mistress again."

"What shall I call you?" Thalia whispered, dazed.

"Call me what a friend would, Thalia, for you've been my friend since we were children. This villa where we enjoyed such happy companionship has made me realize . . ." Dia could scarcely go on, so much feeling did she have for this woman and this moment. She took a deep breath, for she wanted to say all that was in her heart.

"I've learned so much this past year. I've learned that *family* is not necessarily defined by blood, but by caring. And I learned how important you are to me, my dearest friend, when I thought you were going to die and be gone from me forever. You know, I never had a sister, but if God gave me a chance to choose one, I would choose Thalia."

Tears shone in Thalia's dark eyes and spilled over. Dia hugged her, tears dancing in her own eyes. Aunt Grata dabbed at hers with a napkin; no one on the portico was unaffected. The slaves had halted in their tasks, fascinated, envious, watching one of their own receive her freedom.

Dia, her arm around Thalia, turned her to face the other women.

"Thalia is freed. Most Noble Imperial Princess Galla Placidia declares it." She smiled at Thalia, sweeping her hand to include the other dinner guests. "And you could ask for no greater witnesses—two royal houses for you, Thalia; no less would do."

Thalia flushed crimson. Abashed to find herself the center of attention, dazzled and thrilled and feeling as if she were dreaming,

Thalia dipped her head toward the others and groped for her chair. Aunt Justa stood, raising aloft her gilt-edged wineglass.

"To Thalia," Justa said warmly. "We always considered you one of the family, dear."

Dia joined the others in drinking a toast to the freedwoman, and Thalia, who had lived with royalty all her life and understood protocol, managed somehow, despite her racing heart, to accept the honor with as much grace as if she had been a princess.

By now the unexpected and joyful occasion had warmed the women toward each other, raising their spirits and loosening their tongues more surely than strong wine. The aunties, being naturally gregarious, had no difficulty keeping the talk flowing. The subject came around to families.

"I believe in family," declared Justa. "It's having that tie, that comforting knowledge that you always have someplace you belong. I know what you're thinking, Dia, but kinship isn't entirely meaningless. Now I know perfectly well you weren't speaking of Grata and me in your pretty speech—by the way, excellent speech, my dear; I was quite moved—"

"Oh, yes," cut in Grata, "we know *exactly* who you meant— certain unmentionable persons of the *other* side of the family—"

"Honorius, for one," Justa slipped in. "What on God's green Earth your father was thinking when he named that boy Emperor I'll never—"

"That Serena, for another. She always reminded me of a wicked witch." Grata turned to Singledia and Winnifreya and confided, *"Dreadful* woman, simply dreadful; you wouldn't believe—"

"Oh, we heard all about it, dear," Justa went on, "the petition and everything. The people will prevail, you know. This was once a Republic, after all. Don't feel badly. Why, your grandmama Justina would have fed Serena to the bears *years* ago. Mama could get quite a temper up—"

"So could Papa. He kept bears—"

Dia lost the thread of the conversation, smiling to herself. The mention of the bears uncannily drew her mind back to surprising Atawulf in the bath, when she imagined he was one of Grandpapa's bears. Everything, it seemed, reminded her of Atawulf.

She looked at Thalia. Even in the midst of freeing her friend, she had a fleeting vision of Atawulf, for it was during that night in the garden, watching the fireflies, that the idea first came over her. The memory made her eyes mist; blinking rapidly she pulled herself together and held onto the thread of conversation.

Winnifreya confided to Dia that she had misjudged the Roman princess when they first met, but that she was not sorry to have made her acquaintance. Dia's heart ached for Winn, whose world had darkened with Alaric's death, but the queen seemed to be emerging into life again. She felt the healing magic of the villa, too, and she drew nourishment from the peace which wrapped the land like mist.

Winn was saying to Dia, "We're given only one moment in which to live, only *this* moment is ours. 'Tis what we find in each moment, and in each other, that makes our lives. If we miss each other . . ." Winnifreya touched Dia's arm. "Trust your heart, that's what I'm trying to say. Aye, I feel a need to tell you that, Placidia—trust your heart."

Dia nodded, a choking lump in her throat. She didn't know what her heart was saying right now. She didn't know which to trust, the evidence of her eyes or the yearnings of her soul.

After-dessert wine in hand, Justa took Singledia traipsing through the garden to look at the flowers and have a heart-to-heart. Grata led the young ladies across the footbridge and under the pavilion, telling them tales of emperors and captured queens. "Zenobia was held prisoner here, Queen of Palmyra. Of course, the kindly Emperor eventually set her free so she could marry a nobleman. A neighbor . . . oh, it was terribly romantic . . ."

Winn, Dia, and Thalia wandered around the moat talking quietly of past journeys. Later, after everyone met again in the shade of the portico, Singledia came to Dia and Thalia. She congratulated Thalia and told Dia she had something to say to her, and that she hadn't spoken up before because Atawulf would be beside himself if he thought his mother involved herself in his affairs.

"My son is an honorable man, Placidia. I don't believe he deceived you."

"But the document . . ."

"Atawulf is also proud, and sometimes foolish, but I know a young woman every bit as proud and foolish. No human being on Earth is perfect, and that's including the both of you. Atawulf may have made a mistake, but you misjudge him, Galla Placidia. You must realize that, or you do not know my son."

Dia shook her head. "I thought I did." She soon bade Singledia good evening, for she could bear the subject no longer.

Then, on the way back through the garden, Aunt Justa linked her arm in Dia's and said conspiratorially, "Singledia promised to speak with him tomorrow. She agrees with me—holding you hostage is not the answer."

She should have been elated by the news, but somehow it seemed a hollow victory in the still of the empty garden.

The garden was empty, quiet, dark, and it should have felt peaceful, but peace eluded Atawulf. He gazed up at the canopy of stars, and he wondered if peace was an illusion, like a dream you couldn't hold, and he wondered why looking into infinity felt so lonely.

He had grave decisions to make, did the king, and he liked none of the choices.

Sigeric had thundered in with riders, reporting a scout's story that two legions from the east were disembarking at Ravenna—hardened troops from the Persian frontier, rumor said. Going after Atawulf, rumor said. Spearheading an attack, not to roust the Goths from the villa, but to exterminate them.

Aye, the king had hard choices to make.

He could stay and fight, but it would be a tough, bloody fight, a multitude of deaths, and the hollow eyes of wives and mothers, brothers and sons.

And how long could the Goths hold out, encircled by thousands, protecting a country villa from two seasoned legions? No, he could not give them death. Or slavery.

He knew what he must do. A king must lead his people to peace, toward life, hope.

They would move out—again. He had made sure they were prepared; they could be ready in a day. Sunrise after tomorrow, the Goths would be on the road. It would be hard, tearing themselves away from sanctuary. But the people were rested now, healthy and hearty, their bodily wounds healed, their spirits lifted and renewed; it would be a good journey.

He drew his eyes down from the stars and looked toward the pale glow of lamplight illuminating Dia's curtained window.

Which brought him to the next decision he had to make this night. What to do about Dia. Take her into flight with him? She was right. What real justification could he find for dragging her from home again?

The truth? That he couldn't bear the thought of letting her go, knowing if they parted now, their lives would never touch again?

Would she even believe him?

And if he did say those words, what was he offering her? Life on the move, on the run, with fortunes so precarious that the Goths could end up homeless, hungry, and hunted.

And here were her aunts, begging to take her home.

Only a fool would hold on to her.

Only a fool believed he could hold love captive, keep love by force.

He wrestled with that fool for long, painful moments, staring silently up into the lonely wastes of the night. A gentle whiff of honeysuckle wafted on the night breeze, and he saw the fireflies winking and darting in the black garden.

They only shine when they're free, he remembered Dia saying. He knew what he had to do.

Atawulf strode down the peristyle to face the hardest moment of his life. He had sent word this morning; Dia would be expecting him, and he wasn't sure what he was going to say.

First his mother, and then his sister, had cornered him already. His sister was growing strange. "Trust your heart," was all she said. His mother had said more. She told him what he already knew: that he couldn't hold love against its will. But she also told him that if he had words hidden in his heart unspoken, he had best speak them now or carry their burden the rest of his life.

Dia awaited him on the private balcony, for her aunts were unaccustomed to being roused at such an early hour. When Atawulf appeared in the doorway her heart leapt. She had cried herself to sleep last night, and now she hoped this moment would be the answer to her prayers. He would tell her it was all a mistake, that she was wrong; he would show her that the tender lover that night in the pavilion, in the garden, was the true Bold Wolf, the man who loved her.

She wanted to forgive and be forgiven, but he had not spoken. How did she know which Atawulf to believe?

Atawulf had slept only in the short hours before dawn, and the corners of his eyes were shadowed with hard decisions and long thinking.

Aye, and this was hard, too, being this close to her, with those searching eyes watching his. He turned away from her and leaned upon the balustrade, staring across the garden to the vine-cloaked wall.

"Two legions have landed at Ravenna. From the East." His voice sounded abrupt and harsh in his ears.

Silence stretched behind him as the implication of his words slowly sank in.

"Oh," she finally said, her voice small and quavering.

"We've been up since first light, preparing and packing supplies. At dawn tomorrow we'll be going . . ." He let that hang in the silence.

"Oh." Barely a whisper.

He spun to face her then and said the hardest words he had ever spoken.

"I'm letting you go." His eyes held hers a lingering moment, then he turned his gaze away again, his words rushing relentlessly on. "You may leave with your aunts. In fact, you'd best leave today, by afternoon, and be well on your way before . . . before we move out."

She stood speechless, watching his rigid back, the taut play of muscles as he braced to hear her reply.

"I see," she said faintly.

" 'Tis what you wanted, isn't it?"

"I . . . it's so unexpected, so sudden. I . . . you're leaving? Where will you go?"

"North and west, into Gaul. We're getting out of your precious Italia; maybe Honorius will be content with that. I assure you, my people have no wish to see Italia again." He stared into the sky, thinking of foundering ships, deathly fevers, shallow graves—and of Alaric.

"I've had little joy in it," he said softly.

Dia looked away.

He turned to look at her now as she stared at the top of the wall, at the future. Her silhouette, almost close enough to touch, made his soul cry, but he let his eyes memorize her features: the delicate dark fringe of eyelashes, the dainty turned-up nose, the graceful curve of her throat, those full lips begging to be kissed. Her chin trembled; quickly she bowed her head.

"I wish . . . I wish your people Godspeed."

"Do you?"

"Of course. You know I feel . . . close to them." *But do you know how I feel about you?* her eyes pleaded as she turned to him, but he was lost in some thought of his own.

Leave it alone, Atawulf, he told himself brutally. *Let her go. Don't make it harder by saying things she doesn't want to hear.*

But what had been between them hovered there, hummed in the air.

I loved you. The words were there, on the tip of his tongue, and he would say them now, before they went unsaid forever.

The doors onto the balcony burst open and Sylvanus hurried through.

"Majesty!" the old man gasped. "One of your captains is beating my stablemaster with bit and bridle. Captain Sigeric, it is, and he's going to kill him!"

Atawulf glared ferociously at the steward, then his gaze darted hopelessly toward Dia. Her face was pale, frozen in defeat and regret. With savage effort he tore himself away and bounded down the balcony steps, crossing the garden at a run.

He isn't coming. Dia stood in the midst of the courtyard, waiting as their baggage was being loaded into the carriages. Her longing glances could find him nowhere in the milling courtyard.

Their good-byes were said; friends among Goths and slaves gathered to see them off.

Then the baggage was loaded, the carriages were ready, and Aunt Justa said they'd have to be getting on if they were to reach their nearest friends before nightfall.

He isn't coming. Dia sought him one more time before stepping up into the carriage and sitting beside Thalia, facing her aunts in the plush interior. She sat stiffly, trying not to peer out the windows; startled, she jumped when Priscus Attalus appeared at her window.

"I wish I were going with you, nobilissima."

"I wish you were, too, Priscus."

"I fear if I did, the Emperor would have my head."

"Yes, I'm afraid so. I'll speak to my brother for you, tell him it was all a misunderstanding."

"I . . . I'm sorry, Princess . . . about letting you down."

"Yes, I know."

"I really wouldn't have gone along, you see, except that I thought . . . I thought it wouldn't do to interfere in matters of the heart. And if you don't mind my being so presumptuous, I was under the impression that you loved him. Forgive the confusion of a tired old man's brain, but the problem seems rather, well, childish in the extreme."

Priscus Attalus nodded and slapped his hand on the window ledge. "Well, now, I'm holding you up. I imagine you're eager to return to court and leave off all this wandering. I'll be on the highway tomorrow with the Goths, and I must admit I envy your safe passage home. Good-bye, Princess."

Dia laid her hand briefly on his. "Good-bye, Priscus Attalus."

He backed away and waved at the driver; the carriage rolled forward, horses' hooves clattered on the flagstones—a lonely sound of sad departure—and Dia looked back, knowing it was she who envied Priscus his journey with the Goths.

He isn't coming.

The carriages rumbled out the gates, with their retinue of private guards before and behind. As the walls dwindled and disappeared behind a bend in the tree-shaded avenue, Dia sank back into the plush cushions. She felt as if she were leaving behind everything green and alive and real in her life. *Mother of God, why am I doing this?* If Atawulf loved her—and she believed, oh, yes, she believed he did—then she was a queen of fools. And if he didn't love her—either way she was a queen of fools.

She blinked. Her aunties were watching her, keen-eyed. Abruptly she thrust her head out the window.

"Stop the carriage! Stop at once!"

The driver looked undecided, slowing the horses.

"You will stop this carriage now!"

Something in her tone reminded him that this was an Imperial Princess leaning out the carriage window shouting at him like a wild woman. He slowed the carriage to a rocking halt.

"Turn around. I'm going back."

"Yes, nobilissima."

He carefully guided the carriage between the trees and made a wide circle through the pasture back to the road. Dia leaned back, her heart pounding. This was madness, but she was doing it.

Thalia beamed at her, and Aunt Grata said to Aunt Justa, "I knew she'd make the right decision."

"*You* knew? Grata, *I* told you."

As the carriage rounded the bend, heading back for the gate, they met a flash of red and gold as Atawulf galloped at them on Red Demon. He passed them, his face a study in astonishment. Dia thrust her head out the window.

"Oh! Stop the carriage!"

The driver rolled his eyes and leaned back on the reins. This time he brought the horses more easily to a standstill, but not before Demon had already reared and circled and trotted back to the carriage window.

Atawulf grinned through his beard.

"Forget something, Your Royalty?"

"Yes," she answered breathlessly. "Did you?"

"Aye. Come out of that carriage, woman." He dismounted, his clear blue eyes never leaving hers.

"Is this an abduction, Bold Wolf?"

"Is this an invitation?"

She opened the carriage door. "Oh, aye, it is."

She stepped to the ground, and they stood close enough to feel the pull. His eyes spoke, filled with the sight of her, and his fingers reached for her, touched her hair, her temple, cheek, and lips—parting lips, breath-quickened.

She started to speak, but she let her heart speak, her eyes speak, and he bent his head and kissed her.

She soared in his kiss, then she twined her fingers in his hair, glared up at him, and said fiercely, "You'll never be free of me, Bold Wolf."

Then, to distant cheers and whistles and wolf-howls from the

Goths on the wall, Atawulf flung back his head and laughed that great soul-shaking laugh of his. He swung her about in a circle and enfolded her in strong arms, arms that clearly said they never meant to let her go.